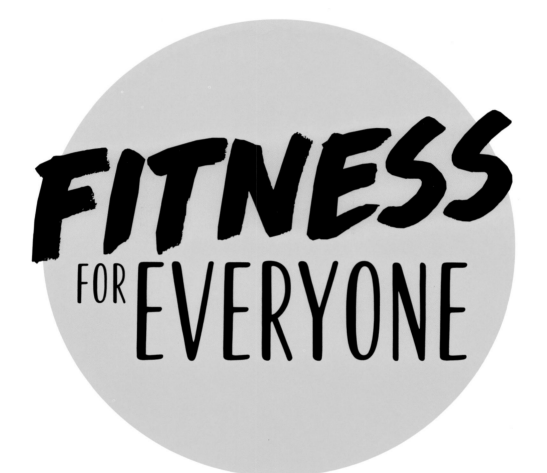

FITNESS
FOR EVERYONE

50 EXERCISES FOR EVERY TYPE OF BODY

>>> LOUISE GREEN <<<

ALPHA

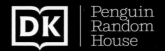

Publisher Mike Sanders
Editor Christopher Stolle
Senior Designer Jessica Lee
Art Director William Thomas
Photographer Joanna Wojewoda
Proofreaders Georgette Beatty & Lisa Himes
Indexer Louisa Emmons

First American Edition, 2020
Published in the United States by DK Publishing
1450 Broadway, Suite 801, New York, NY 10018

Copyright © 2020 by Louise Green

Copyright © 2020 Dorling Kindersley Limited
DK, a Division of Penguin Random House LLC
20 21 22 23 24 10 9 8 7 6 5 4 3 2 1
001-319226-DEC2020

ISBN: 978-1-6156-4899-3
Library of Congress Catalog Number: 2020941363

DK books are available at special discounts when purchased in bulk for sales promotions, premiums,
fund-raising, or educational use. For details, contact: DK Publishing Special Markets,
1450 Broadway, Suite 801, New York, NY 10018
SpecialSales@dk.com

Printed and bound in Canada
Photo Credits: Cover 123RF.com: Liliia Rudchenko / rudchenko; Dreamstime.com: Shakila Malavige.
All other images © Dorling Kindersley Limited

For the curious
www.dk.com

CONTENTS

FOREWORD

I remember the first time I stepped into a gym. It was back in 2012, right after my doctor called me fat and told me I was going to die.

Fueled by anger and defiance, I walked into the gym for the first time since I had graduated from my undergrad program in 2009. It was embarrassing and awkward. I didn't know how to use the equipment. I felt like I was in everyone's way. On top of that, I wasn't thin, white, or wealthy. It felt like standing under a spotlight right when I wanted to disappear.

That first day, I didn't even work out. I just moved from machine to machine and watched other people get their sweat on. I left feeling ashamed and defeated, thinking there's no way I can do any of this stuff.

I went home and tried to search the web for exercises specifically for people in larger bodies. The results shocked me. All I found were people who didn't look like me demonstrating exercises I knew I couldn't do. I hired a trainer, but they didn't know how to work with a plus-sized client. I decided it was time to teach myself: I fired the trainer and I started reading everything I could find.

The journey was long and difficult. More than once, I felt like a lab rat in a maze as I tested exercise theories and modifications on myself. It paid off. I slowly started to find fitness and confidence, which led me to trying other physical activities. That's how I discovered my true passion: running. I've run eight marathons since then, including the four I finished in 2019. I covered every single mile with the full power of my 300-plus-pound body.

I'm living, breathing, running proof that fitness isn't one-size-fits-all. It doesn't look like what the media, magazines, and influencers portray it to be. The truth is, "fit and healthy" looks different on everybody. Fitness belongs to all of us. It's our birthright—that's the beauty of it.

Standing in that gym on Day One of my personal fitness journey, I'd have given anything for a book like *Fitness for Everyone* and a trainer like Louise Green. She's a masterful trainer and has an intuitive understanding of what folks' bodies are capable of.

This book couldn't have come from anyone but her—and it couldn't have come at a better time. The health and fitness industry is beginning to shift, but work like this is a much-needed antidote for the diversity and inclusion it's still missing.

Each exercise Louise details here has variations for people of all shapes, sizes, body types, and abilities. It gives us all the equal opportunity to receive the benefits of getting our bodies moving, even if we don't look like someone on the cover of a magazine. (Let's be real here: Who actually does?)

I can't express what it means to me—and the culture as a whole—that *Fitness for Everyone* depicts representations of what human beings who exercise actually look like. Thumbing through, you'll surely see someone you can identify with.

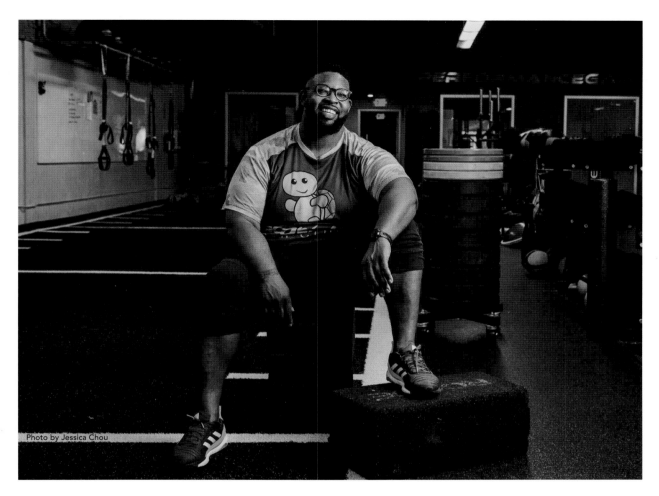

Whether you've been working out for years or you're just getting started, you'll find something new, challenging, and exciting.

The best part is that Louise's teachings don't require you to change who you are or to wait for when your body is thinner, fitter, or more stronger to get going. That's a damn gift.

Learning to personalize and modify my fitness routine all those years ago helped me make peace with my body and changed my life. I became more physically fluent. I got stronger mentally and physically.

Fitness for Everyone can help you learn these things and come into your own athletic abilities too. This book will empower you, inspire you, challenge you, and change you. All you have to do is turn the page and start your next chapter.

MARTINUS EVANS
(Instagram: @300poundsandrunning)

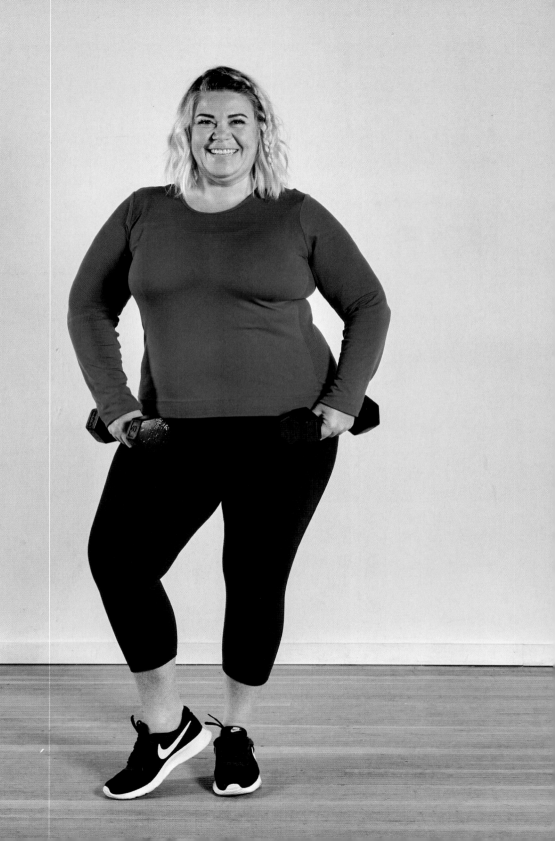

YES, YOU *CAN* EXERCISE!

As a young girl, I was very active. I grew up in the 1970s and 1980s. As kids, most of our free time was spent in the great outdoors using our imagination and channeling it to physical play. In addition to free-play physical activity, I also participated in organized sports. I played on the school teams for basketball, volleyball, and track and field, and on weekends, I played in a soccer league.

Even at a young age, I loved how exercise made me feel: invigorated and alive. It was a place I could lose myself for an hour or two and push myself to my limits. What I know now is that I loved the endorphins and the chemical change in my brain when I exerted my body. Now I see that exercise, even at that young age, made me a happier, more confident kid and fostered a strong foundation for mental and physical health into my teen and adult years.

Through my 20s, I lived through a period of extreme diet culture. As many young women do, I got caught up in the idealistic beauty standards presented in our media message and I wasn't accepting of my body. I used exercise as a tool to achieve my thinness goals and it started to taint my joy for movement.

On yet another quest to lose weight, I decided I'd give running a try. I figured that if all the runners on the front of magazines were lean, I could be too. On the first night of my new running clinic, I was terrified but was completely taken aback to learn that my new run leader was a plus-size woman. She was the first plus-size athletic representation I'd ever seen.

Her name was Chris and I trained with her for more than 12 weeks to the 5K finish line. She trained me like an athlete, never once mentioning my body size or the limitations I thought I had. Chris profoundly changed my life. I ran that 5K race, then many 10K races, then half-marathons, then transitioned into triathlons. I cycled long-distance events. I stopped dieting and started believing in myself at the size I was and started living my athletic dreams in the body I had. I eventually left my career to pursue fitness full-time to show others that no matter what they think their limitations are, they can still enjoy the power of physical movement.

Maybe your struggle isn't weight, but whatever it is, accepting and adapting to how your body moves is absolutely possible. Meeting Chris made me realize that if one person can impact me so greatly with the power of her representation, then what would the world be like if fitness magazines and health and wellness bookshelves accurately represented the population at large? What if people of all ages, abilities, sizes, and ethnicities were included? What would the impact be if representation was commonplace and normative bodies became all bodies?

I believe representation is the gateway to accessibility and, ultimately, global health and wellness. This book is dedicated to the people who long to see themselves in fitness and who long to be inspired and motivated by a likeness of themselves. Representation shows us what's possible.

I hope this book shows you that fitness is possible in your life.

LOUISE GREEN
(Instagram: @louisegreen_bigfitgirl)

LOUISE GREEN

I'm a person who tenaciously goes after my goals and dreams. I want to live fully and I never want stereotypes to define who I am and how I should live. I care about people deeply. I have the skill to genuinely empathize with each person I meet and take time to see life through their lens. On a personal level, the benefits to exercise have profoundly changed my life from a physical, mental, and spiritual position. Fitness has fostered better body confidence and leadership and has allowed me to expand my mind to believing that almost anything is possible. I believe that everyone should have access to these benefits.

For more than 15 years, I've worked diligently to listen, observe, and adapt fitness for my clients—many of whom have felt unrepresented and sidelined by our fitness culture. Together, we've found ways to make things work and created options for them to adapt the same mindset and fortitude to achieve their goals. Diversity and inclusion of people of all walks of life are essential to the betterment of humankind. Everyone deserves to be seen and considered so we can all enjoy the benefits of health and wellness.

Fitness has changed who I am. I'm a more confident, body-positive, adventurous, and less fearful person than I was before. I've trained for some pretty rigorous goals, and fitness has taught me that if I show up and engage in the process with a positive mindset, I'll succeed. Not everyone's body is the same and we all have different capabilities, but we all have goals we can take higher—no matter our size, age, or ability. I became consistently active in my late 20s and I've always been someone who has enjoyed a variety of movement: running,

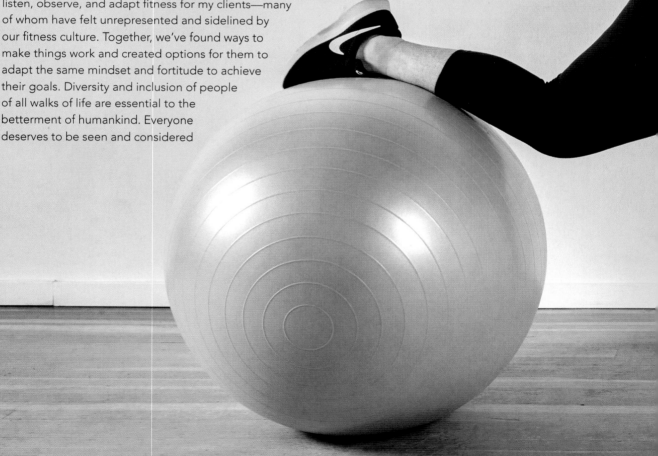

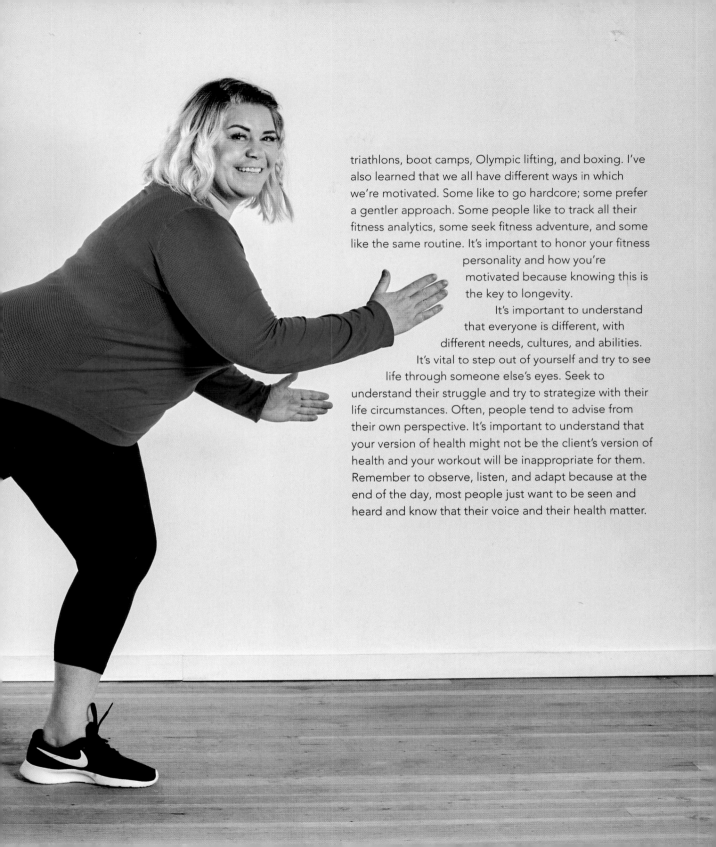

triathlons, boot camps, Olympic lifting, and boxing. I've also learned that we all have different ways in which we're motivated. Some like to go hardcore; some prefer a gentler approach. Some people like to track all their fitness analytics, some seek fitness adventure, and some like the same routine. It's important to honor your fitness personality and how you're motivated because knowing this is the key to longevity.

It's important to understand that everyone is different, with different needs, cultures, and abilities. It's vital to step out of yourself and try to see life through someone else's eyes. Seek to understand their struggle and try to strategize with their life circumstances. Often, people tend to advise from their own perspective. It's important to understand that your version of health might not be the client's version of health and your workout will be inappropriate for them. Remember to observe, listen, and adapt because at the end of the day, most people just want to be seen and heard and know that their voice and their health matter.

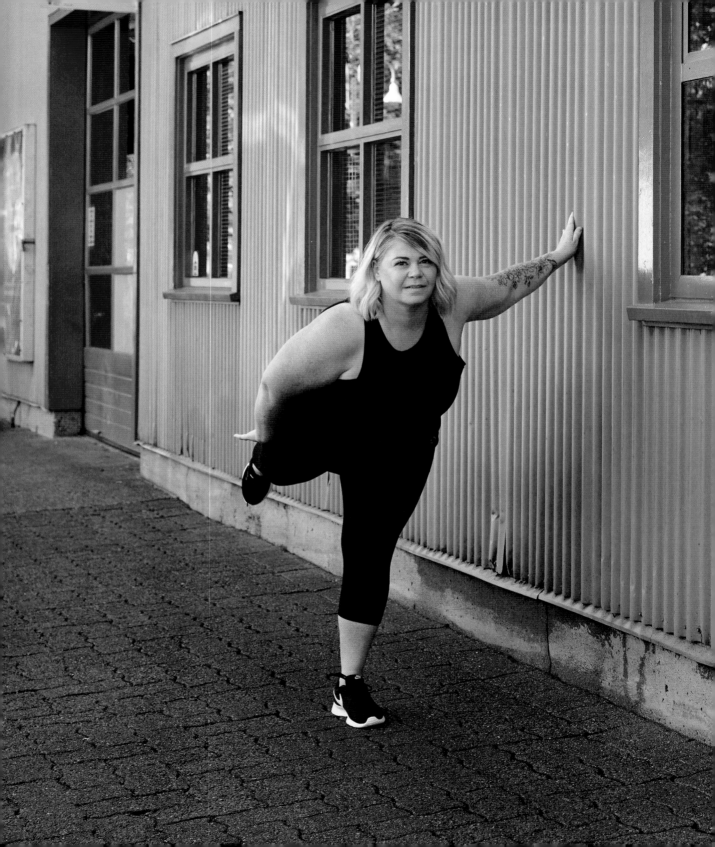

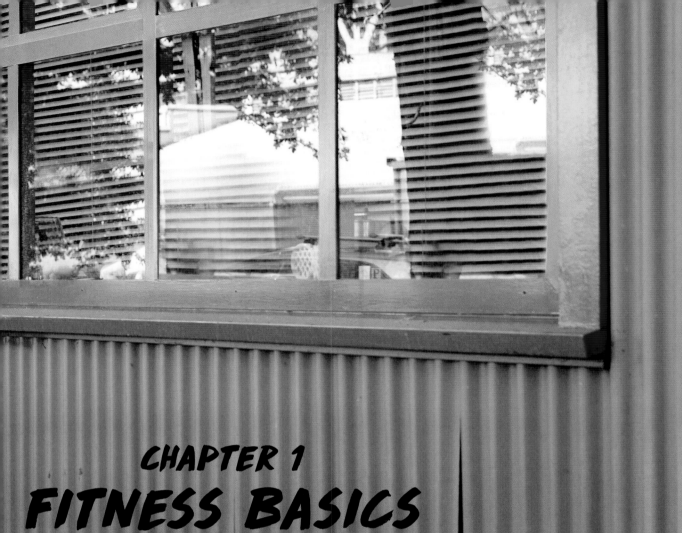

CHAPTER 1
FITNESS BASICS

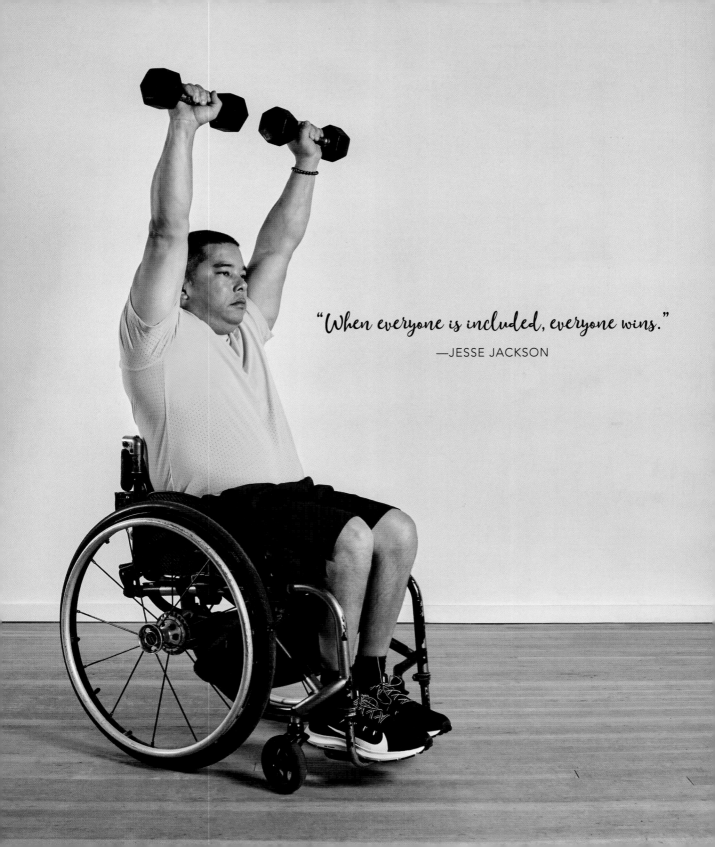

"When everyone is included, everyone wins."

—JESSE JACKSON

MAKING FITNESS ACCESSIBLE— FOR EVERYONE

Fitness is for *every* body. People sometimes feel excluded from fitness culture because they don't see someone like themselves. Representation removes barriers and invites *everyone* to join. This book will show you how fitness can benefit your daily life— no matter your shape, size, age, or ability.

BOOST SELF-ASSURANCE.

One of the biggest reasons people don't exercise is because it can look intimidating. But there's more than one way to perform an exercise and still gain similar benefits. The variations and modifications in this book will help you slowly build confidence and strength. Starting slowly not only cultivates body trust but is also the safest method to increase strength without injury at a rate that's doable for your body and your mind. When and if you're ready, you can move to a different variation or modification or even try the main exercise.

IMPROVE MENTAL HEALTH.

Exercise can elevate your mood and help you manage mild to moderate depression, anxiety, and stress. Exercise releases endorphins that flood your brain with chemicals that make you feel good. Exertion can help you feel like a new person. Things that bothered you before working out might no longer be major concerns. Making exercise accessible to all people means equity in access to wellness for the body but also the mind.

DEVELOP BODY CONFIDENCE.

When you feel strong in your body, you often have higher body confidence. The more you rely on your body, the more you trust it—and with trust comes higher confidence. This is the case for all bodies of all abilities. If you stop believing in your body, you lose confidence. Strength training and overall physical conditioning are important because with growing confidence, we're more inclined to try new things and set new goals. Body confidence is the forward momentum to physical achievements because you can trust you're capable.

INCREASE STRENGTH, BALANCE & ENDURANCE.

Physical fitness is important at any age but particularly as you grow older. Optimal fitness supports lasting independence and allows you to say yes to life without worrying your body will fail you. Daily movement creates better mobility and strength training builds muscle mass and bone density. Plus, there are all the physiological benefits exercise can bring, such as managing blood pressure as well as reducing the risk of heart disease, diabetes, and high cholesterol. Daily exercise also aids in better sleep, balance, and overall endurance to manage life with more vigor and ease.

ENHANCE THE QUALITY OF LIFE—NOW & ALWAYS.

It's sometimes difficult to imagine the importance of quality of life and the "golden years" when you're young, but exercise can lay the foundation for aging well. Exercise can even slow down the aging process. People who have a lifelong history with exercise show less decline in muscle and bone density loss as opposed to those who didn't exercise. Regular exercisers also often have elevated immunity. The benefits of fitness are really endless, but living independently with a great quality of life for as long as you can is a great motivator to move regularly.

MAKING FITNESS "CORE" IN YOUR LIFE

If you're new to fitness and wondering how this book can help you,
there are some things you might want to know before starting:
why you're doing something, what the benefits are, and how to be effective.
You'll also want to know how to set goals and take safety precautions.
What follows are the different components of fitness and their methodology.

BUILD MUSCULAR STRENGTH.

Muscular strength is all about creating strength within the muscles by increasing demand on the fibers. You can achieve this strength by performing exercises with your body weight, resistance bands, weight machines, and dumbbells. Putting demands on your muscles breaks down muscle fibers. Then your body builds muscular strength when your body repairs this breakdown. In time, increasing loads with lower reps will develop muscular strength. With this book, you can work on the strength routines, and over time, you can increase the weights to achieve improved muscular strength.

INCREASE MUSCULAR ENDURANCE.

Muscular endurance is the ability to put your muscles under demand for longer periods. Muscular endurance comes with longer training periods and specifically with weight training that involves higher reps and lighter weights. This conditions the muscle fibers to work under demand and helps you endure longer workouts. Muscular endurance is also achieved in long-distance training, such as cycling and running. With this book, you can achieve muscular endurance by performing the longer workouts, and when the time is right, you can stack workouts at the back of the book.

DEVELOP CARDIOVASCULAR ENDURANCE.

Cardiovascular endurance relies on how efficiently your heart, capillaries, and lungs work together to supply oxygen to your lungs. The more practiced you are in cardio fitness, the more efficiently this system runs—and you can thus perform cardio exercise for longer periods. At first, you might feel out of breath, but over time, the more you push this system with each workout, the more you can do cardio fitness with ease. With this book, you can improve cardiovascular endurance by choosing the longer interval workouts.

IMPROVE FLEXIBILITY.

Flexibility is an important part of fitness because without it, your muscles can shorten, and over time, this can cause biomechanic challenges and occasionally injury. Working on flexibility will improve your range of motion and make movements easier. With this book, you can improve your flexibility by performing the stretch and balance routines.

SEEK MEDICAL APPROVAL.

If you've been away from fitness for a long time or things have changed in your health, it's a good idea to let your doctor know about your new fitness plan. Getting approval from a doctor will set you up for the best safety and, of course, the best success.

START SLOWLY & LIGHTLY.

Many people like to go back to what they were once able to do and start there, but our bodies evolve over time and we must respect where we are today.

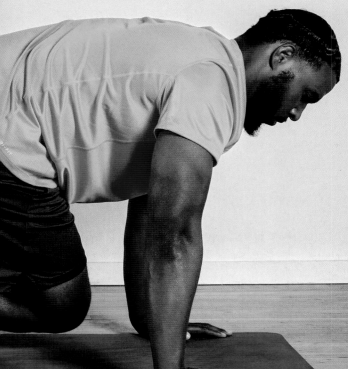

Starting slowly and lightly is responsible fitness, and once that feels good, you can slowly increase your weights and elevate your intensity.

HAVE PROPER FOOTWEAR.

Make sure you have good footwear that's designed for exercise. You can open yourself up to injury if you don't protect your feet with shoes that work for movement. Talk to your salesperson about athletic training shoes, cross-trainers, or gym shoes.

UNDERSTAND YOUR RATE OF PERCEIVED EXERTION.

This is a tool for trainers to understand how hard their clients are working, but if you're exercising alone, this is a great way to gauge your own intensity.

- **1: Very light activity:** anything other than sleeping or watching TV

- **2 to 3: Light activity:** feels like you can maintain for hours; easy to breathe and hold a conversation

- **4 to 6: Moderate exercise:** breathing heavily; can hold a short conversation; still somewhat comfortable but becoming noticeably more challenging

- **7 to 8: Vigorous activity:** borderline uncomfortable; can speak a sentence

- **9: Very hard activity:** very difficult to maintain exercise intensity; can barely breathe; can speak only a few words

- **10: Max effort activity:** feels almost impossible to keep going; completely out of breath; unable to talk; can't maintain for more than a very short time

For this book, the 4 to 6 range is a great goal to work toward. You might find yourself in the 7 to 8 range if you're performing the interval workouts with cardio bursts, but moving beyond this can be unsafe. Knowing where you are and how you're supposed to feel is the ideal way to self-regulate your exercise routine.

CREATING CONSISTENCY & CONFIDENCE

Regular fitness requires planning, intention, and daily motivation. Exercising often cultivates energy, and when you establish at-home routines, you eliminate some of the obstacles. Plus, with the key tips discussed here, you'll set yourself up for success.

START SLOWLY.

Being patient and listening to your body are essential to longevity in fitness. It doesn't matter what you could do 5 years ago or 20 pounds ago. All that matters is now. Many people do too much too fast and end up injuring themselves. Smart fitness means going slowly, feeling successful with every workout, and then incrementally moving up to bigger challenges. Starting slowly also builds body trust and confidence as well as helps you prevent potential injury.

SET A GOAL.

Setting goals is a great way to not only develop a fitness routine but also to maintain that routine. Write weekly and monthly goals where you can see them every day. Having a plan—and working on that plan—creates confidence in the process. One great way to establish goals is to use the SMART method:

- **Specific:** I want to work out at least three times a week by performing two interval workouts and one stretching session.
- **Measurable:** Through these workouts, I want to increase my weights 1 to 2 pounds per week.
- **Attainable:** I need to set a goal that's doable. Yes, I can work out 7 days a week, but this isn't attainable or sustainable over time.
- **Realistic:** My goal must be realistic and something I can sustain over time given all my other responsibilities in life.
- **Timely:** I'm going to do this for 30 days and then reassess my goals.

MAKE SCHEDULES.

If you fail to plan, then you plan to fail. This is never more true than with exercise. If you're waiting for the right moment or a free moment, life takes over and you never end up exercising. You must intentionally make time to look after your health and wellness. Once a week, get out the calendar and make appointments with yourself to move. If something important comes up, this appointment is rescheduled, not cancelled. Honor your health and make time to move, move, move.

CREATE THE SPACE.

Making exercise easy and accessible to attain will lead to longevity in your commitment. If you have a space created just for your movement and some basic equipment, then you're setting yourself up for success. Make this space a place you want to be, add some motivational posters, and get a speaker for listening to music. Make this space your own because this area will play a significant role in your motivation.

DO WHAT YOU LOVE.

Some exercises are difficult and not the most fun, but a difference exists between enduring a difficult movement for a minute or two and doing a movement you really dislike. If you don't like something, you're likely to give up easily. When you first start a fitness routine, the conditioning phase can present quite a challenge—mentally and physically. Give a certain workout a chance for a week or two before you decide whether you like it. Find workouts you enjoy because they're the gateway to consistency and sustainability.

BREATHING TECHNIQUES

When it comes to exercise, effective breathing can result in efficient performance. The more you move, the more oxygen you need. But it's not just how much you move. You also need to consider the type of physical movement you're performing and which breathing style best supports that.

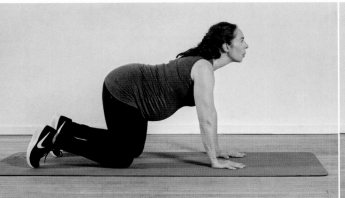 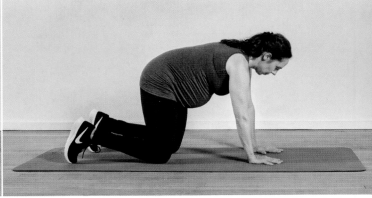

WEIGHT LIFTING

When weight lifting, inhale at the moment of least resistance and exhale at the moment of most exertion. For example, when performing a shoulder press, exhale when you raise the weights toward the ceiling. Then inhale as you lower the weights to your shoulders. Over time, as you lift heavier weights, exhale with more force.

CARDIOVASCULAR

There are some different schools of thought on cardio breathing. I recommend my clients to nose breathe to a certain point, then to mouth breathe when things get more intense. Deep breathing, no matter where it's coming from, will help oxygenate the muscles and carry you through the workout longer. For example, when running in place, for every two to four strides, you should breathe in and out. When you first start running in place, inhale and exhale through your nose with every two movements. When you increase the intensity, inhale and exhale through your mouth with every two movements. (Even though this book includes a wide variety of cardio moves, try to maintain a full breath for every two symmetrical or near-symmetrical movements.)

STRETCHING

Breathing properly while stretching can greatly enhance your flexibility. Inhale slowly through your nose as you go into a stretch, expanding your belly. Exhale slowly through your nose or mouth as you release the stretch. Inhaling as you find your way into the stretch and exhaling as you're deepening into the stretch make the stretch more intense but also more effective. For example, with a side bend, with your arms raised toward the ceiling, inhale as you bend your torso to your left and reach as far as you can with your right hand. Exhale as you hold this position and deepen into the stretch by leaning in an inch or two more.

ISOMETRIC & BALANCE

Many people hold their breath during isometric (static) and balance exercises. But keeping a steady flow of oxygen into the body makes an exercise more effective. For example, as you find your way into a plank and hold that position, breathe in deeply into the belly and breathe out steadily. This helps you maintain balance while ensuring you continue to get needed oxygen to the muscles that are helping you stay in the plank.

WHAT YOU NEED TO EXERCISE

You can perform every exercise in this book just about anywhere and with minimal equipment. Here are some items you might need to do the main exercises in this book as well as the variations.

YOGA MAT

Because there are a lot of exercises performed on the floor, you might want to have a mat underneath you. Look for ones that will accommodate your height, can prevent slipping, and have ample cushioning.

CHAIR

Chairs can help with issues of limited mobility or flexibility. Find one that's sturdy and feels comfortable.

RESISTANCE BAND

Buy a resistance band that's at least 10 feet long and has comfortable handles. It should be made from high-quality rubber or have a ruffle cloth cover.

CLOTHES

You should wear clothes that allow you to move freely and without constriction. What matters most is that you feel comfortable no matter what you wear.

WALL

You can find a wall anywhere. They offer accessibility, stabilization, and resistance—and they can even aid in relaxation. Use one with plenty of nearby floor space.

BOLSTER

You might find you feel more comfortable performing some exercises and variations with a bolster under your legs or other body parts. Find one that feels comfortable when you hug it to your chest.

WEIGHTS

Start with small handheld weights. In time, when these don't provide the resistance you desire, you can move up to heavier weights.

STABILITY BALL

Finding the best stability ball is as easy as actually sitting on one before you buy it, but also check the weight capacity. You'll want to make sure you feel comfortable and stable while using one.

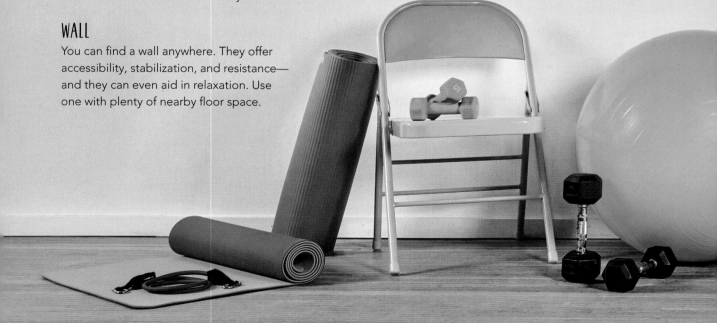

HOW TO USE THIS BOOK

This book has four main components:

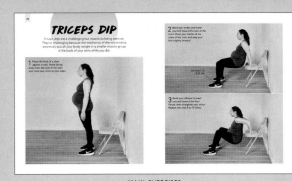

MAIN EXERCISES

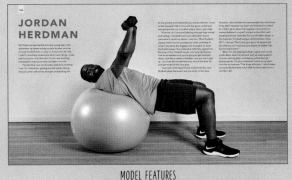

VARIATIONS

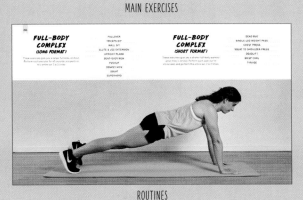

ROUTINES

MODEL FEATURES

MEET THE MODELS

LOUISE	SIMI	THEA	JORDAN	FAEDRAGH	TAZ	ROB
READ HER STORY ON PAGE 10.	READ HER STORY ON PAGE 64.	READ HER STORY ON PAGE 106.	READ HIS STORY ON PAGE 146.	READ HER STORY ON PAGE 180.	READ HIS STORY ON PAGE 208.	READ HIS STORY ON PAGE 238.

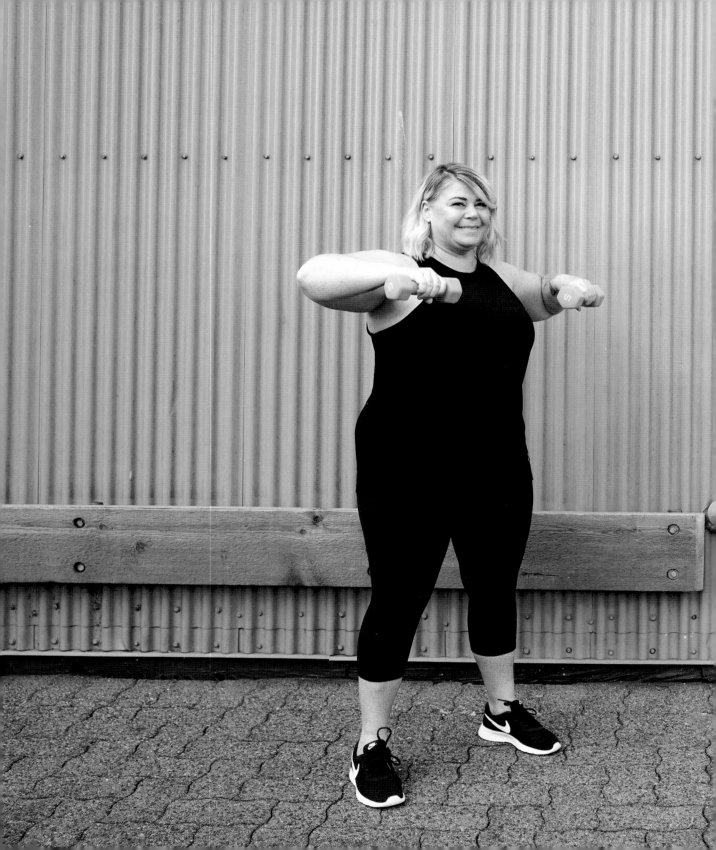

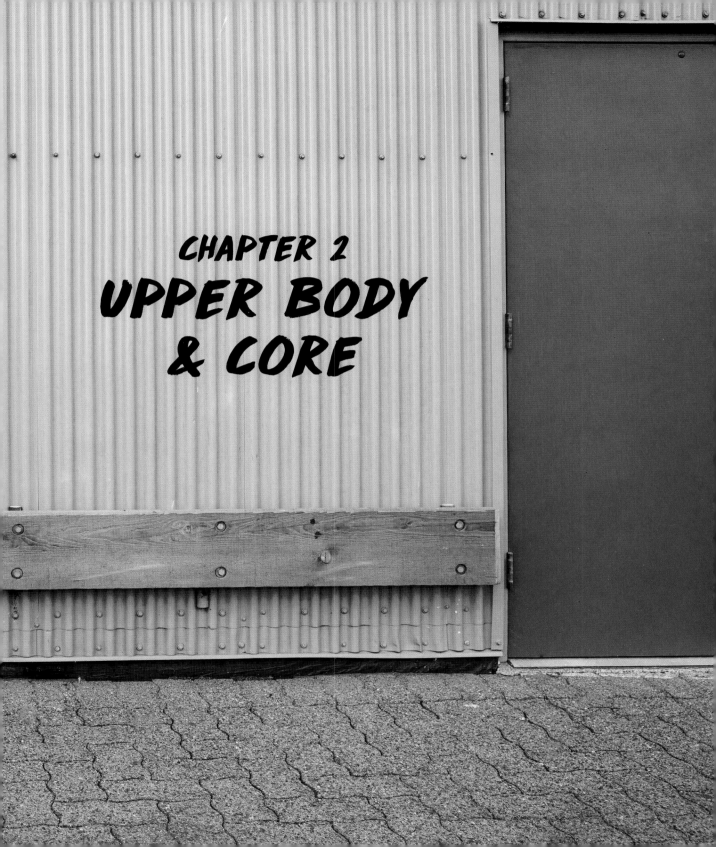

CHAPTER 2
UPPER BODY & CORE

T-RAISE

Strong shoulders are essential for functional everyday living, including lifting, pulling, and throwing. This is a great exercise for using two of the three heads in the deltoids that are critical for these movements: the medial and anterior.

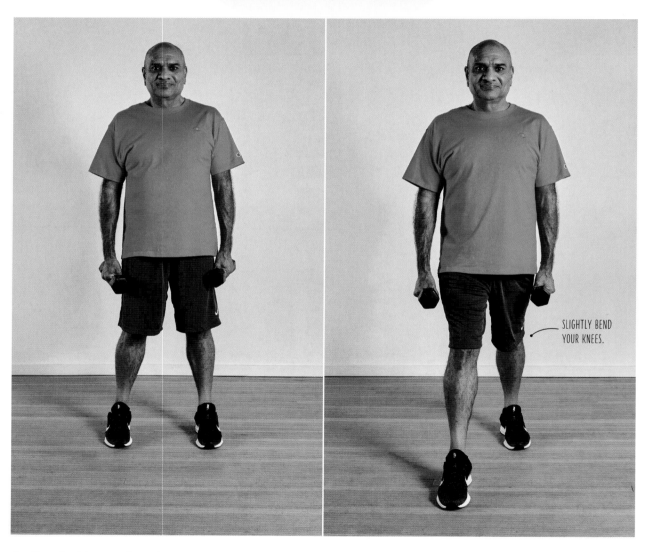

SLIGHTLY BEND YOUR KNEES.

1 Stand with your feet shoulder width apart and relax your arms at your sides.

2 Step your right foot forward until your feet are about 1 to 2 feet apart.

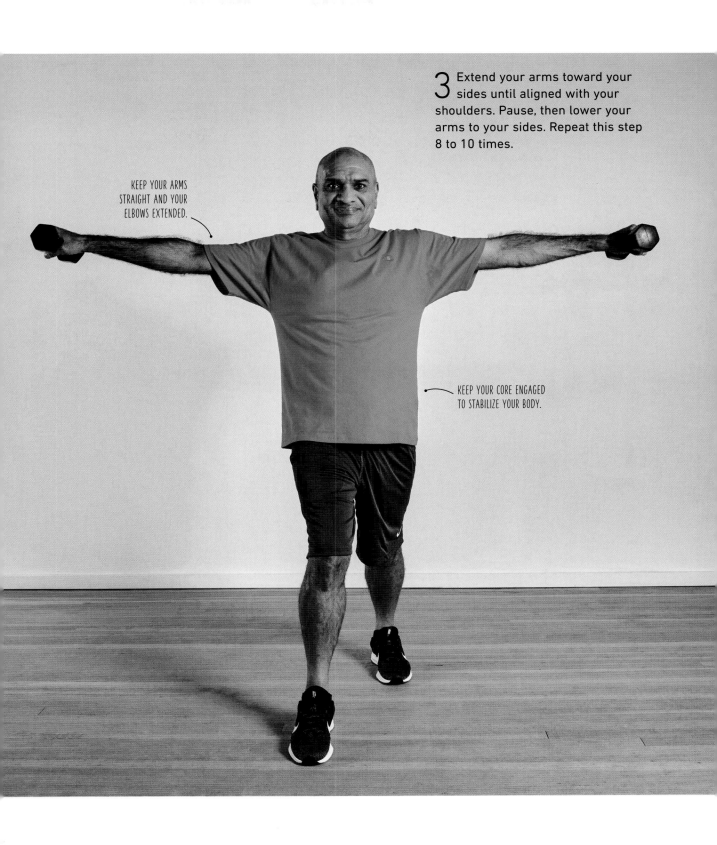

3 Extend your arms toward your sides until aligned with your shoulders. Pause, then lower your arms to your sides. Repeat this step 8 to 10 times.

KEEP YOUR ARMS STRAIGHT AND YOUR ELBOWS EXTENDED.

KEEP YOUR CORE ENGAGED TO STABILIZE YOUR BODY.

// T-RAISE //
VARIATIONS

These modifications offer better stability to allow you to gradually work up to the split stance.

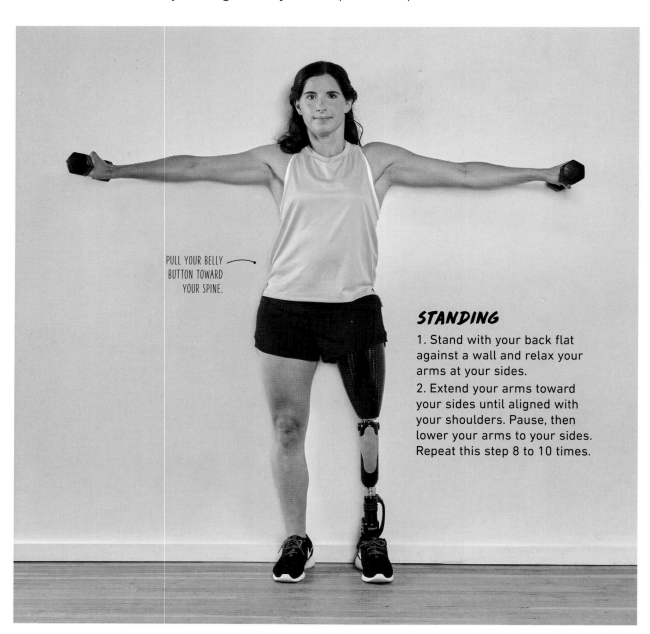

PULL YOUR BELLY BUTTON TOWARD YOUR SPINE.

STANDING

1. Stand with your back flat against a wall and relax your arms at your sides.
2. Extend your arms toward your sides until aligned with your shoulders. Pause, then lower your arms to your sides. Repeat this step 8 to 10 times.

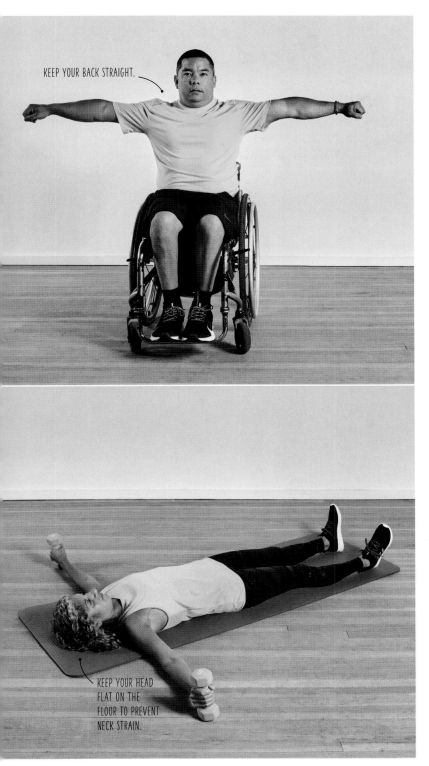

KEEP YOUR BACK STRAIGHT.

KEEP YOUR HEAD FLAT ON THE FLOOR TO PREVENT NECK STRAIN.

SEATED (NO WEIGHTS)

1. Sit in a chair and place your feet flat on the floor under your knees.

2. Extend your arms toward your sides until aligned with your shoulders. Pause, then lower your arms to your sides. Repeat this step 8 to 10 times.

ON THE FLOOR

1. Lie on your back on the floor. Hold a weight in each hand and relax your arms at your sides.

2. Extend your arms to your sides until aligned with your shoulders. Pause, then lower your arms to your sides. Repeat this step 8 to 10 times.

CHEST PRESS

Many everyday movements—maintaining posture, pushing, and embracing—involve the pectoral muscles. Plus, they're critical for different actions in fitness and sports. This chest press is great for building strength in your upper body.

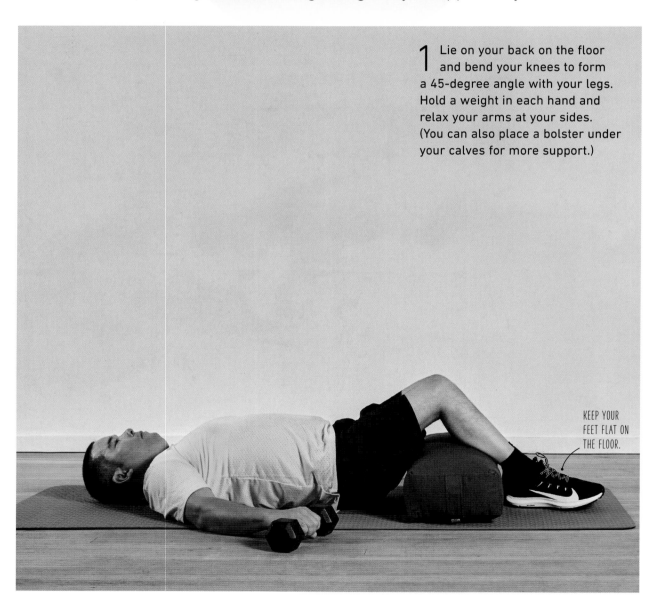

1 Lie on your back on the floor and bend your knees to form a 45-degree angle with your legs. Hold a weight in each hand and relax your arms at your sides. (You can also place a bolster under your calves for more support.)

KEEP YOUR FEET FLAT ON THE FLOOR.

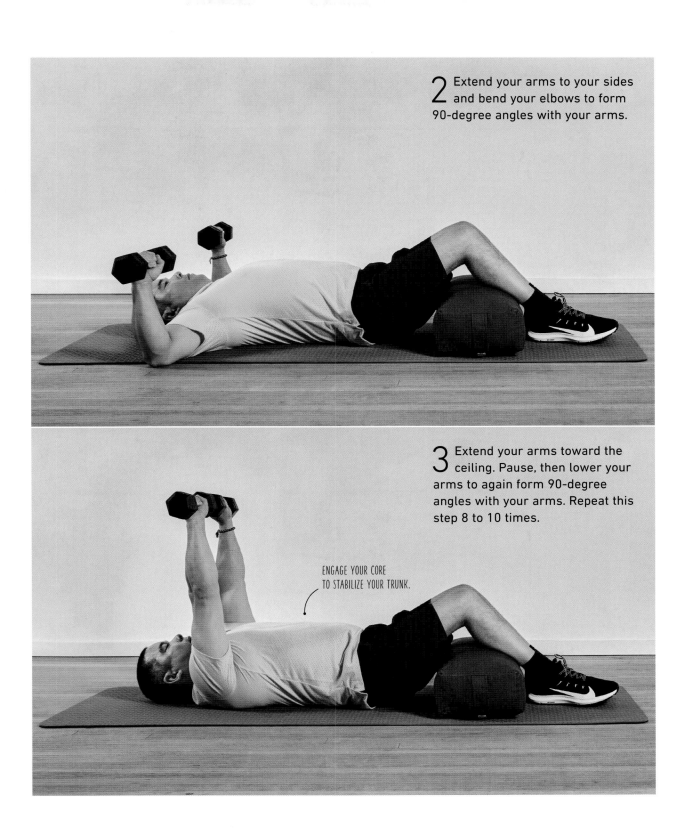

2 Extend your arms to your sides and bend your elbows to form 90-degree angles with your arms.

3 Extend your arms toward the ceiling. Pause, then lower your arms to again form 90-degree angles with your arms. Repeat this step 8 to 10 times.

ENGAGE YOUR CORE
TO STABILIZE YOUR TRUNK.

// CHEST PRESS //
VARIATIONS

These modifications offer variety and options without having to get on the floor or use a bench.

WITH A WALL (NO WEIGHTS)

1. Stand with your back flat against a wall and your feet shoulder width apart. Relax your arms at your sides.

2. Step your feet about 1 foot away from the wall. (Stay closer to the wall if the exercise starts to feel too challenging.)

3. Extend your arms to your sides and bend your arms to form 90-degree angles with your arms.

4. Extend your arms forward until parallel with the floor. Pause, then lower your arms to again form 90-degree angles with your arms. Repeat this step 8 to 10 times.

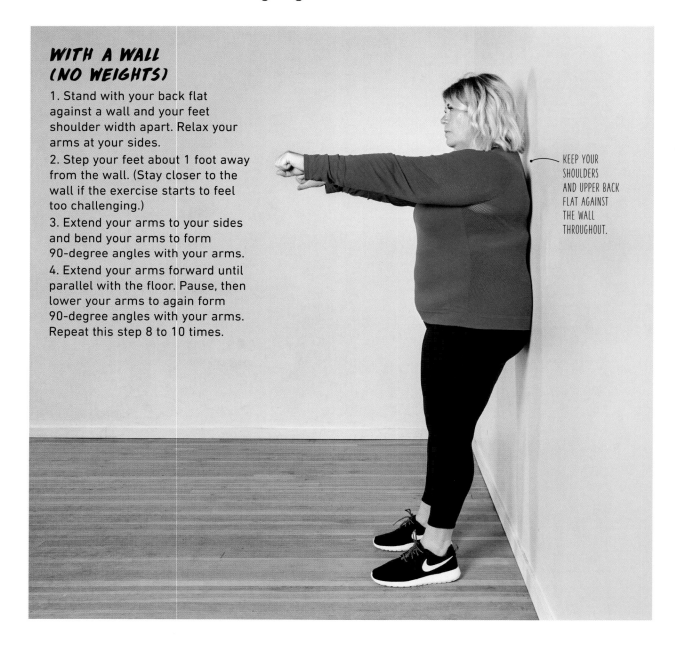

KEEP YOUR SHOULDERS AND UPPER BACK FLAT AGAINST THE WALL THROUGHOUT.

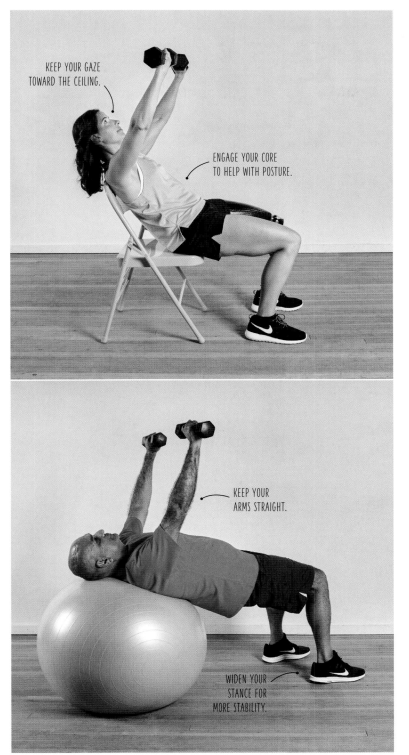

KEEP YOUR GAZE TOWARD THE CEILING.

ENGAGE YOUR CORE TO HELP WITH POSTURE.

KEEP YOUR ARMS STRAIGHT.

WIDEN YOUR STANCE FOR MORE STABILITY.

SEATED

1. Sit on the edge of a seat of a chair and place your feet flat on the floor. Hold a weight in each hand and relax your arms at your sides.

2. Lean backward until your upper back and shoulders are supported by the back of the chair.

3. Extend your arms toward the ceiling until aligned with your lower legs. Pause, then lower your arms to your sides. Repeat this step 8 to 10 times.

ON A STABILITY BALL

1. Sit on a stability ball and place your feet flat on the floor and under your knees. Hold a weight in each hand and relax your arms at your sides.

2. Walk your feet forward until the ball is between your upper back and shoulders.

3. Extend your arms toward the ceiling until aligned with your lower legs. Pause, then lower your arms to your sides. Repeat this step 8 to 10 times.

SQUAT TO SHOULDER PRESS

With multi-joint movements that incorporate different muscles, this exercise offers a full-body experience. These motions take some coordination, but as you get stronger, you can use the momentum of your legs to push through to the press.

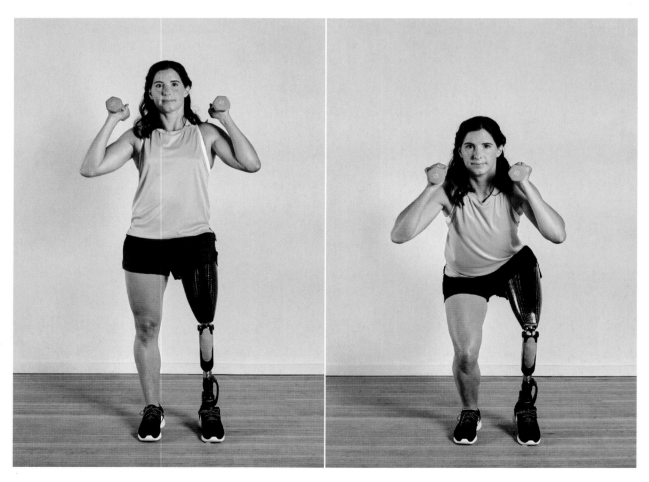

1 Stand with your feet shoulder width apart. Hold a weight in each hand and rest the weights on your shoulders.

2 Put your weight into your heels and bend your knees to slowly lower your body into a squat.

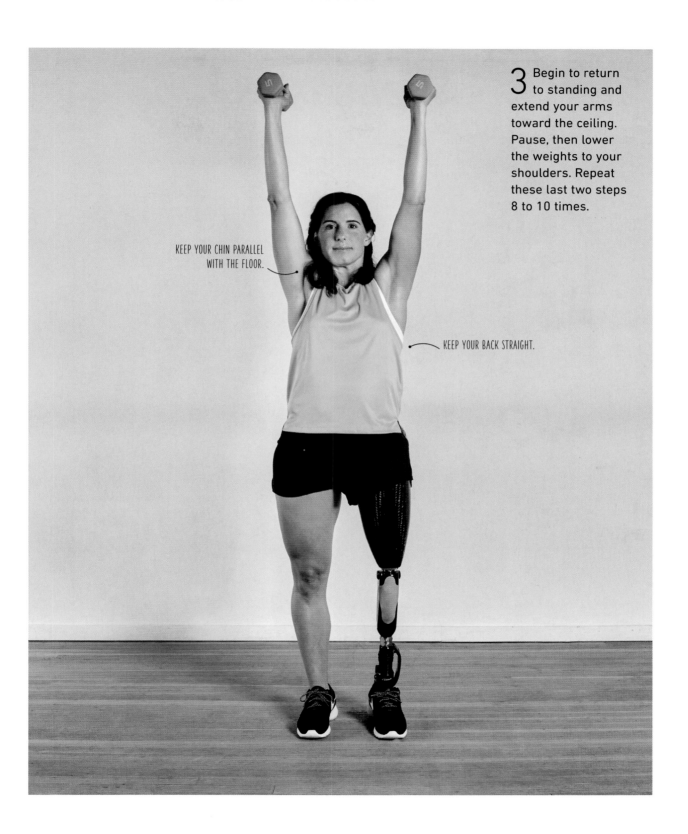

3 Begin to return to standing and extend your arms toward the ceiling. Pause, then lower the weights to your shoulders. Repeat these last two steps 8 to 10 times.

KEEP YOUR CHIN PARALLEL WITH THE FLOOR.

KEEP YOUR BACK STRAIGHT.

// SQUAT TO SHOULDER PRESS //

VARIATIONS

Using the floor or a chair for assistance gives you a variety
of options with less load to slowly build muscle.

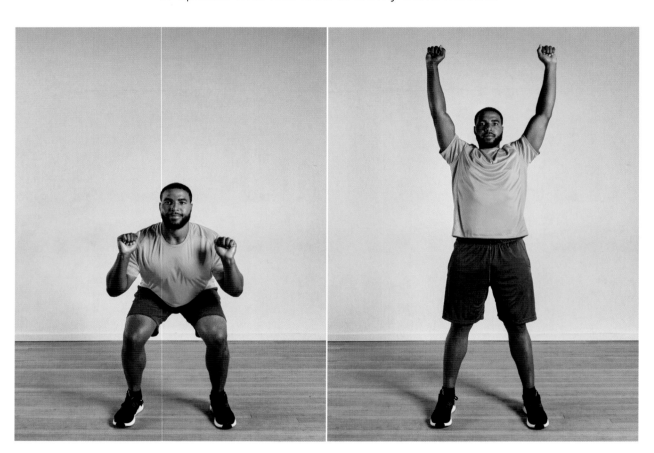

SQUATTING TO STANDING (NO WEIGHTS)

1. Stand with your feet shoulder width apart. Bend your elbows
and form 45-degree angles with your arms.

2. Bend your knees to slowly lower your body into a squat to form
a 45-degree angle with your legs.

3. Begin to return to standing and extend your arms toward the
ceiling. Pause, then repeat these last two steps 8 to 10 times.

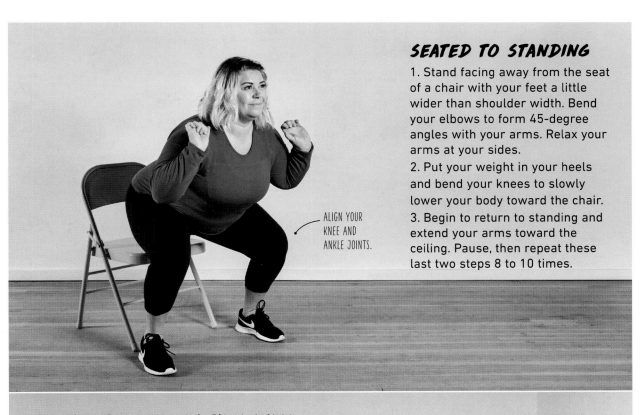

SEATED TO STANDING

1. Stand facing away from the seat of a chair with your feet a little wider than shoulder width. Bend your elbows to form 45-degree angles with your arms. Relax your arms at your sides.

2. Put your weight in your heels and bend your knees to slowly lower your body toward the chair.

3. Begin to return to standing and extend your arms toward the ceiling. Pause, then repeat these last two steps 8 to 10 times.

ALIGN YOUR KNEE AND ANKLE JOINTS.

ON THE FLOOR & WITH A WALL

1. Lie on your back on the floor and place the bottom of your feet flat against a wall. Hold a weight in each hand and rest the weights on your shoulders.

2. Press your feet into the wall and extend your arms over your head until your arms are straight. Pause, then lower the weights to your shoulders. Repeat this step 8 to 10 times.

PRESS THROUGH YOUR FEET TO ENGAGE YOUR GLUTES.

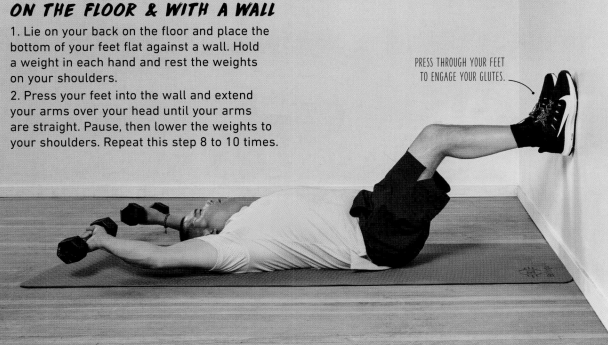

SPLIT STANCE FRONT RAISE

Moving your arms away from your body creates further instability, but forming a split stance with your legs calls on your core to activate for stability. This is technically a shoulder exercise, but you'll work different muscles with each movement.

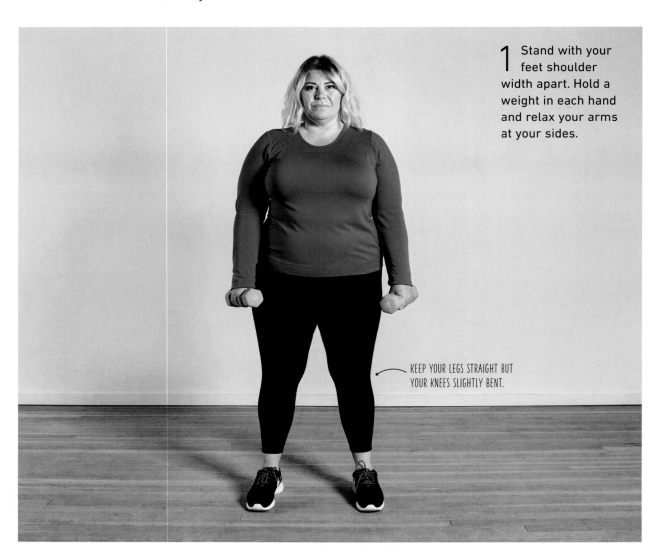

1 Stand with your feet shoulder width apart. Hold a weight in each hand and relax your arms at your sides.

KEEP YOUR LEGS STRAIGHT BUT YOUR KNEES SLIGHTLY BENT.

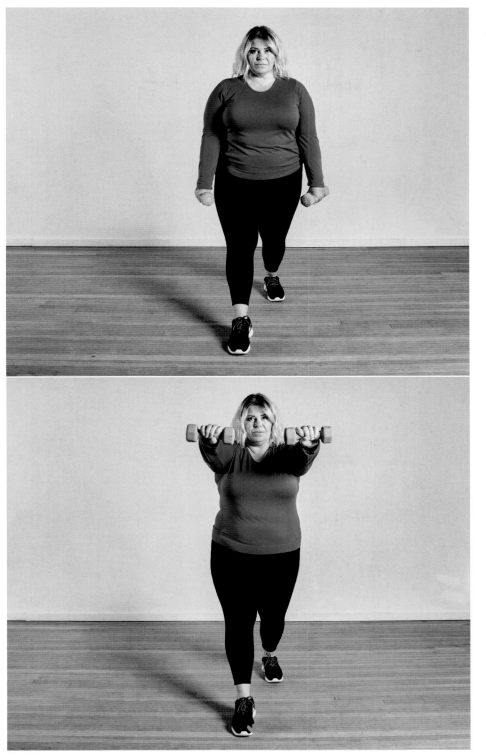

2 Step your right foot forward and place your foot flat on the floor, exaggerating your natural stride by about 2 feet, to form a triangle with your body.

3 Extend your arms forward until aligned with your shoulders. Pause, then lower your arms to your sides. Repeat this step 6 times. Repeat these steps with your left foot stepped forward.

// SPLIT STANCE FRONT RAISE //
VARIATIONS

Doing a split stance puts the body off-center,
but using a chair or a wall can help you ease into the form.

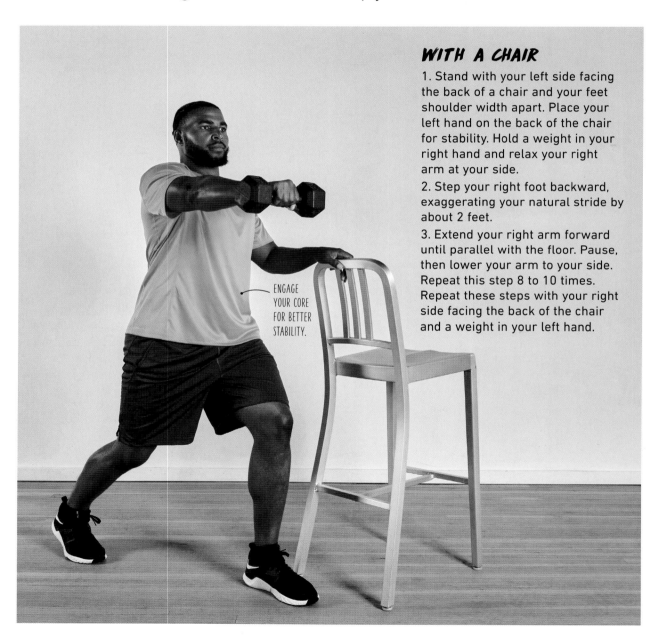

ENGAGE YOUR CORE FOR BETTER STABILITY.

WITH A CHAIR

1. Stand with your left side facing the back of a chair and your feet shoulder width apart. Place your left hand on the back of the chair for stability. Hold a weight in your right hand and relax your right arm at your side.

2. Step your right foot backward, exaggerating your natural stride by about 2 feet.

3. Extend your right arm forward until parallel with the floor. Pause, then lower your arm to your side. Repeat this step 8 to 10 times. Repeat these steps with your right side facing the back of the chair and a weight in your left hand.

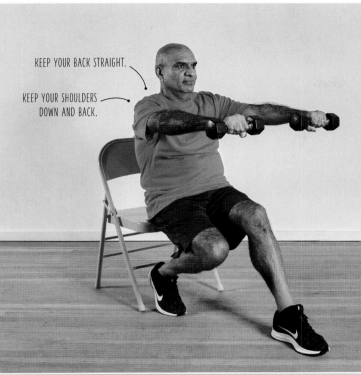

KEEP YOUR BACK STRAIGHT.

KEEP YOUR SHOULDERS DOWN AND BACK.

SEATED

1. Sit on the edge of the seat of a chair. Extend your right leg backward. Extend your left leg forward and place your left foot flat on the floor. Hold a weight in each hand and relax your arms at your sides.

2. Extend your arms forward until parallel with the floor. Pause, then lower your arms to your sides. Repeat this step 6 times. Repeat these steps with your left leg extended backward and your right foot flat on the floor.

WITH A WALL

1. Stand with your back flat against a wall and your feet shoulder width apart. Hold a weight in each hand and relax your arms at your sides.

2. Step your left foot forward and extend your arms forward until parallel with the floor. Pause, then lower your arms. Repeat this step 6 times. Repeat these steps with your right foot stepped forward.

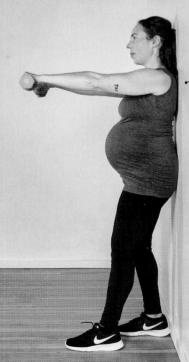

KEEP YOUR SHOULDERS AND BACK FLAT AGAINST THE WALL THROUGHOUT.

PUSH-UP

Push-ups are challenging because you're lifting your entire body weight with the mechanics of your arms and chest. Focus on your form and movements to not only get the most benefits from push-ups but to also prevent injuries.

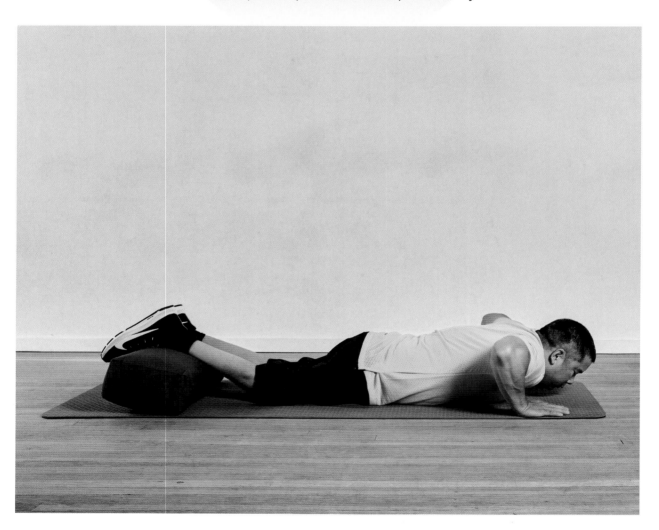

1 Lie on your stomach on the floor. Place your hands and the tops of your toes flat on the floor. (You can also use a bolster to elevate your legs.) Place your hands slightly wider than shoulder width and bend your elbows.

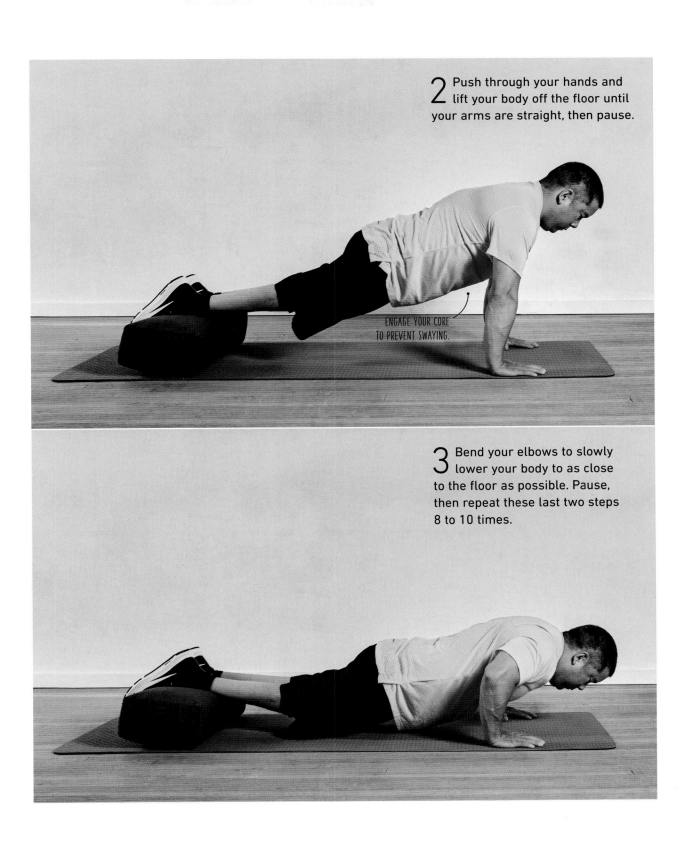

2 Push through your hands and lift your body off the floor until your arms are straight, then pause.

ENGAGE YOUR CORE TO PREVENT SWAYING.

3 Bend your elbows to slowly lower your body to as close to the floor as possible. Pause, then repeat these last two steps 8 to 10 times.

// PUSH-UP //

VARIATIONS

These push-up modifications allow for a more gradual approach to pushing your body weight away from a surface.

WITH A WALL

1. Stand facing a wall with your feet shoulder width apart and relax your arms at your sides.

2. Place your hands flat against the wall and step your feet backward until your arms are fully extended.

3. Bend your elbows to slowly lean your body into the wall until your nose almost touches the wall. Hold this position for 1 second.

4. Push through your hands and lift your body off the wall until your arms are straight. Hold this position for 1 second. Repeat these last two steps 8 to 10 times.

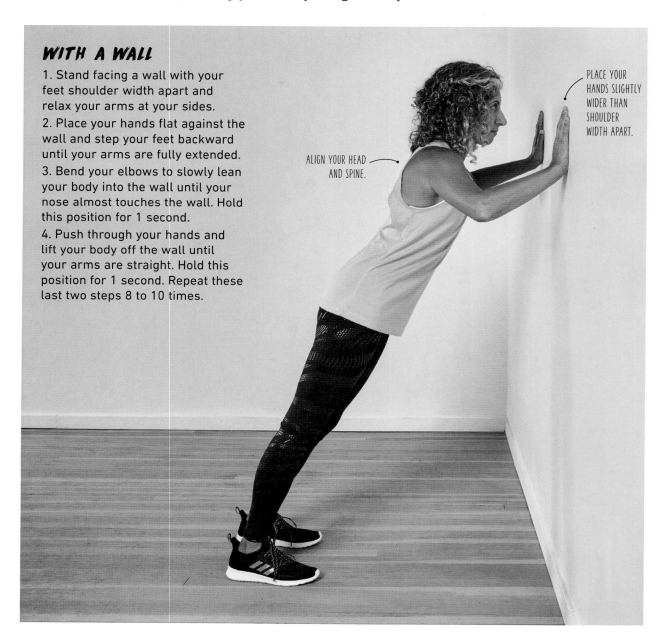

PLACE YOUR HANDS SLIGHTLY WIDER THAN SHOULDER WIDTH APART.

ALIGN YOUR HEAD AND SPINE.

WITH A CHAIR

1. Place the back of a chair against a wall. Place your hands shoulder width apart on the seat of the chair and keep your arms straight. Extend your legs backward.

2. Bend your elbows to slowly lower your body as far as you can toward the seat of the chair. Hold this position for 1 second.

3. Push through your hands and lift your body off the seat of the chair until your arms are straight. Hold this position for 1 second. Repeat these last two steps 8 to 10 times.

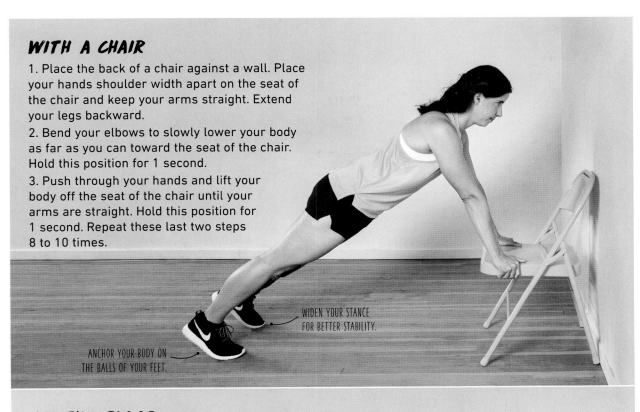

WIDEN YOUR STANCE FOR BETTER STABILITY.

ANCHOR YOUR BODY ON THE BALLS OF YOUR FEET.

ON THE FLOOR

1. Place your hands and knees flat on the floor. Elevate your lower legs off the floor and cross your ankles.

2. Slowly bend your elbows to form a 90-degree angle with your arms and lower your body as far as you can. Hold this position for 1 second.

3. Push through your hands and lift your body off the floor until your arms are straight. Hold this position for 1 second. Repeat these last two steps 8 to 10 times.

ALIGN YOUR HANDS AND SHOULDERS.

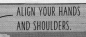

BICEPS CURL CROSSOVER

Who doesn't love strong arms? This exercise is a great way to build bicep strength. Plus, strong biceps make everyday movements like lifting, carrying, and pulling easier. You'll be amazed at how easily you can develop your arms with this curl.

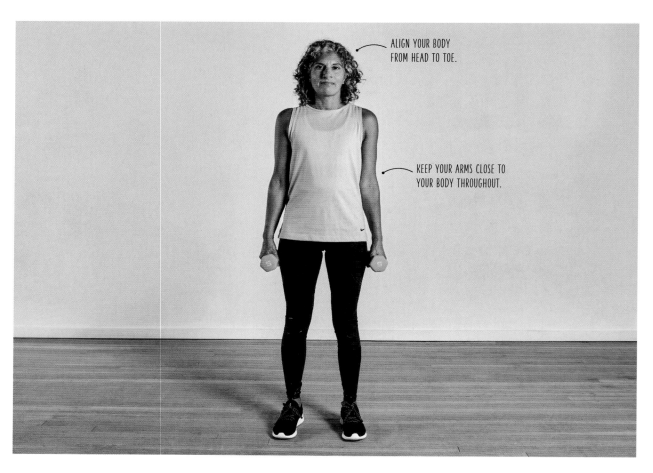

ALIGN YOUR BODY FROM HEAD TO TOE.

KEEP YOUR ARMS CLOSE TO YOUR BODY THROUGHOUT.

1 Stand with your feet shoulder width apart. Hold a weight in each hand and relax your arms at your sides.

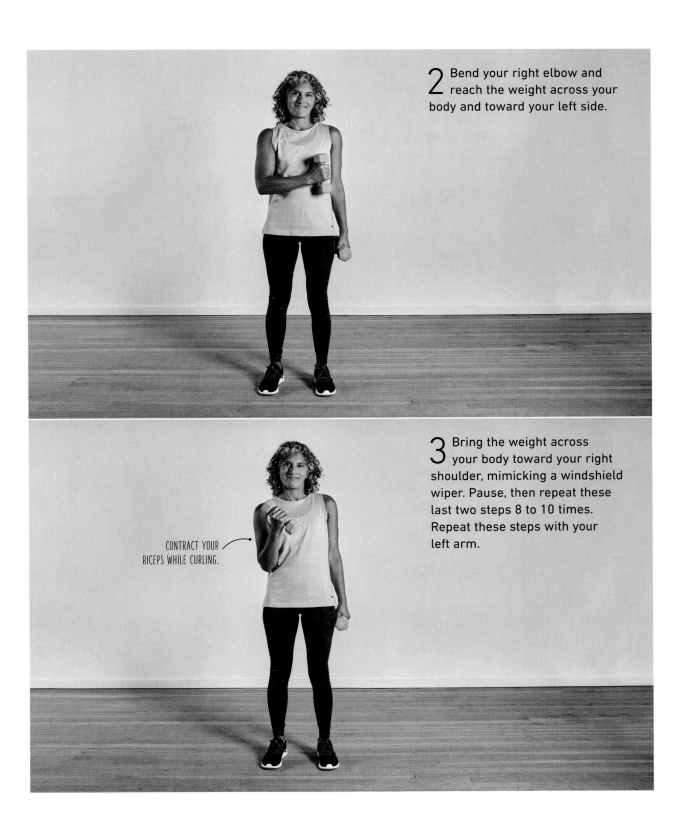

2 Bend your right elbow and reach the weight across your body and toward your left side.

3 Bring the weight across your body toward your right shoulder, mimicking a windshield wiper. Pause, then repeat these last two steps 8 to 10 times. Repeat these steps with your left arm.

CONTRACT YOUR BICEPS WHILE CURLING.

// BICEPS CURL CROSSOVER //
VARIATIONS

These variations offer ways to progress and regress the exercise:
a squat for more challenge and seated for less challenge.

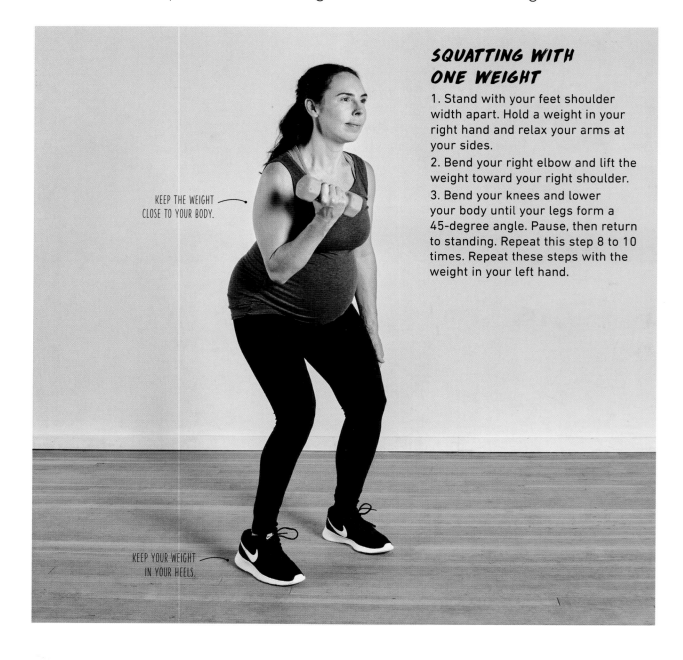

KEEP THE WEIGHT
CLOSE TO YOUR BODY.

KEEP YOUR WEIGHT
IN YOUR HEELS.

SQUATTING WITH ONE WEIGHT

1. Stand with your feet shoulder width apart. Hold a weight in your right hand and relax your arms at your sides.

2. Bend your right elbow and lift the weight toward your right shoulder.

3. Bend your knees and lower your body until your legs form a 45-degree angle. Pause, then return to standing. Repeat this step 8 to 10 times. Repeat these steps with the weight in your left hand.

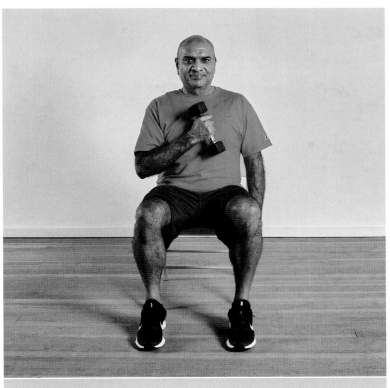

SEATED

In step 1, sit on the edge of the seat of a chair and place your feet flat on the floor. Hold a weight in your right hand and relax your arms at your sides. Continue with the remaining steps.

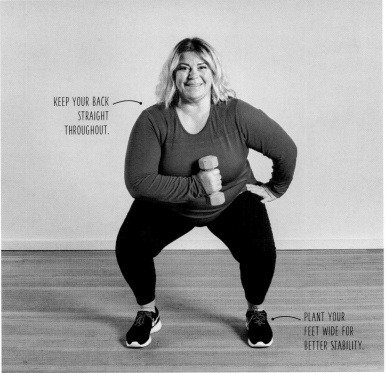

KEEP YOUR BACK STRAIGHT THROUGHOUT.

PLANT YOUR FEET WIDE FOR BETTER STABILITY.

DEEPER SQUAT

1. Stand with your feet shoulder width apart. Hold a weight in your right hand and relax your right arm at your side. Place your left hand on your left hip.

2. Bend your right elbow and reach the weight across your body toward your left side.

3. Bend your knees and lower your body until your legs form a 90-degree angle. Pause, then return to standing. Repeat this step 8 to 10 times. Repeat these steps with the weight in your left hand.

LAT PULLDOWN

Lat exercises can really help with strengthening the torso. When the trunk of your body is strong, you can hold a better posture. When your posture is sound, you tend to have fewer issues with biomechanics and overall body ailments. Strong lats for the win!

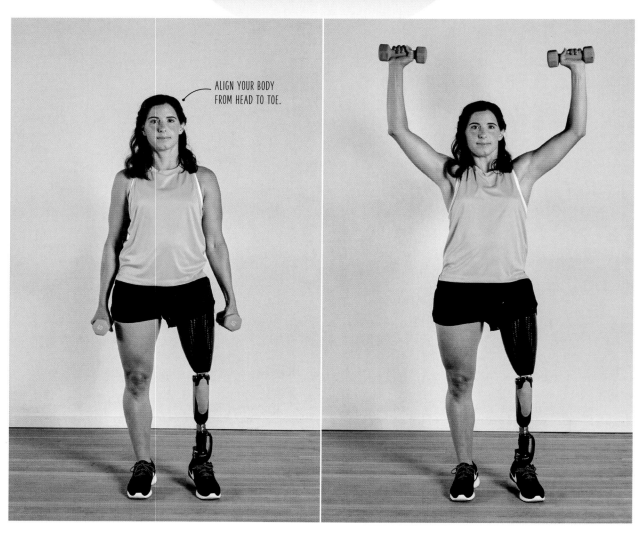

ALIGN YOUR BODY FROM HEAD TO TOE.

1 Stand with your feet shoulder width apart. Hold a weight in each hand and relax your arms at your sides.

2 Extend your arms toward the ceiling and slightly bend your elbows.

3 Slowly lower your arms until the weights align with your shoulders. Pause, then extend your arms toward the ceiling. Repeat this step 8 to 10 times.

ENGAGE YOUR CORE
TO MAINTAIN FORM.

// LAT PULLDOWN //

VARIATIONS

These modifications are great if balance or standing is an issue.
The one with the resistance band offers variety to your workout.

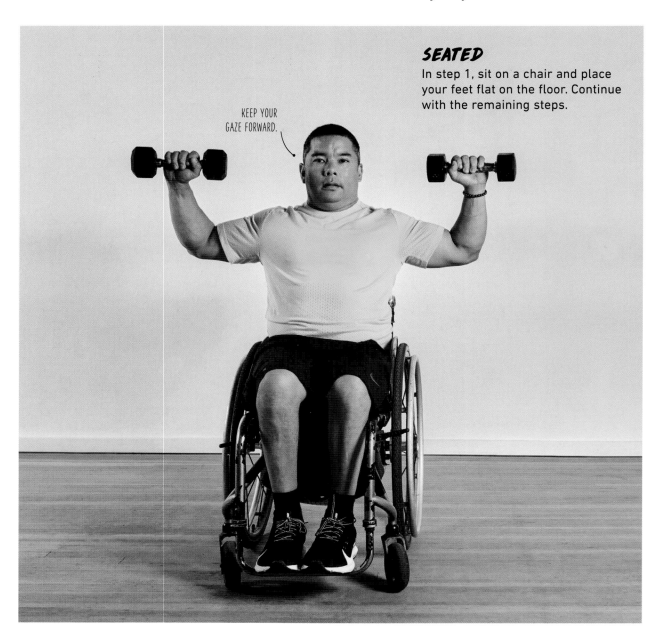

SEATED

In step 1, sit on a chair and place your feet flat on the floor. Continue with the remaining steps.

KEEP YOUR GAZE FORWARD.

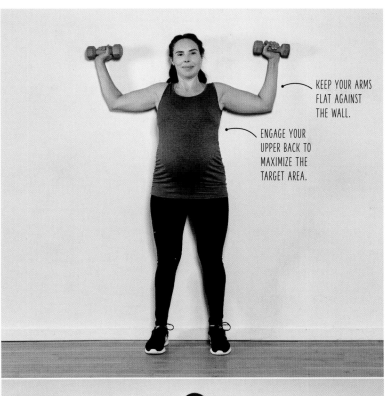

KEEP YOUR ARMS FLAT AGAINST THE WALL.

ENGAGE YOUR UPPER BACK TO MAXIMIZE THE TARGET AREA.

WITH A WALL

1. Stand with your feet shoulder width apart and your back flat against a wall. Hold a weight in each hand and relax your arms at your sides.
2. Extend your arms toward the ceiling and slightly bend your elbows.
3. Slowly lower your arms to form 90-degree angles with your arms until the weights align with your ears. Pause, then extend your arms toward the ceiling. Repeat this step 8 to 10 times.

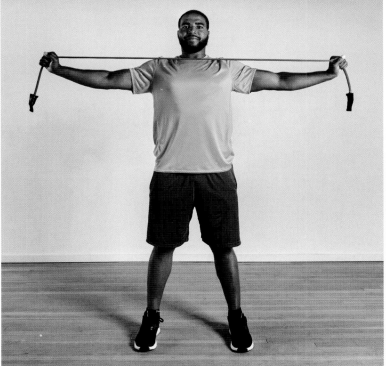

WITH A RESISTANCE BAND

1. Stand with your feet shoulder width apart. Hold a resistance band taut across your chest with your hands.
2. Raise your arms until your hands align with your shoulders. Slightly bend your elbows.
3. Slowly pull the band toward the sides of your shoulders. Pause, then lower the band to your chest. Repeat these last two steps 8 to 10 times.

TRIANGLE PUSH-UP

By placing your hands in the form of a triangle, you can perform
a push-up in a more narrow position than a regular push-up.
This kind of push-up targets your chest but also activates your
triceps, helping build strength in these muscles.

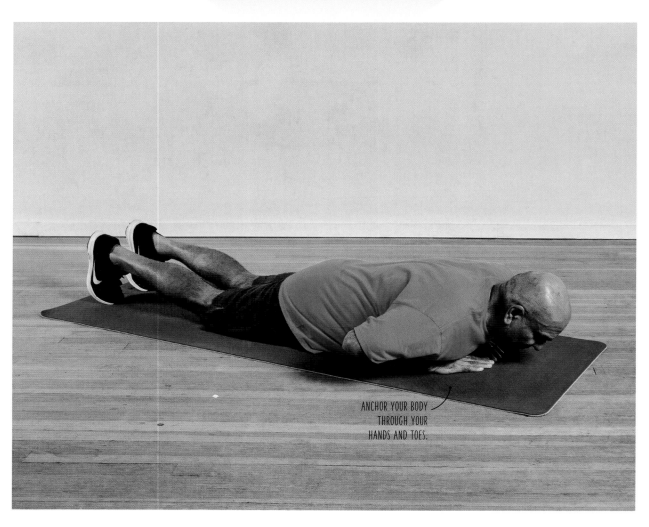

ANCHOR YOUR BODY
THROUGH YOUR
HANDS AND TOES.

1 Lie on your stomach on the floor. Place your
hands and the balls of your feet flat on the
floor. Form a triangle under your chest with your
index fingers and thumbs.

2 Push through your hands and lift your body off the floor until your arms are straight. Hold this position for 1 second.

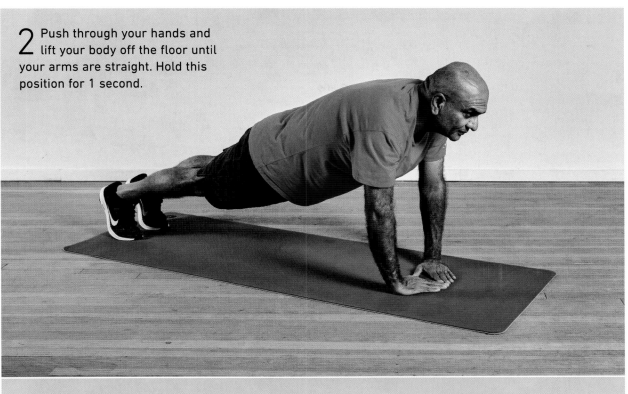

3 Bend your elbows to slowly lower your body to as close to the floor as possible. Hold this position for 1 second. Repeat these last two steps 8 to 10 times.

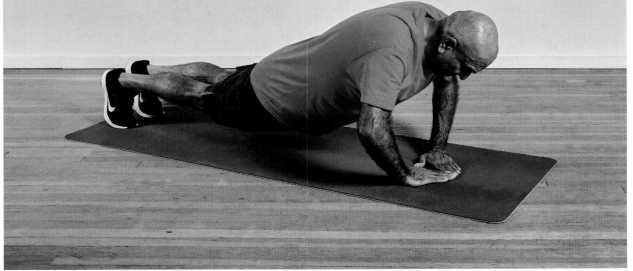

// TRIANGLE PUSH-UP //
VARIATIONS

Performing this exercise on your knees or on elevated surfaces
can help you build strength gradually and then progress.

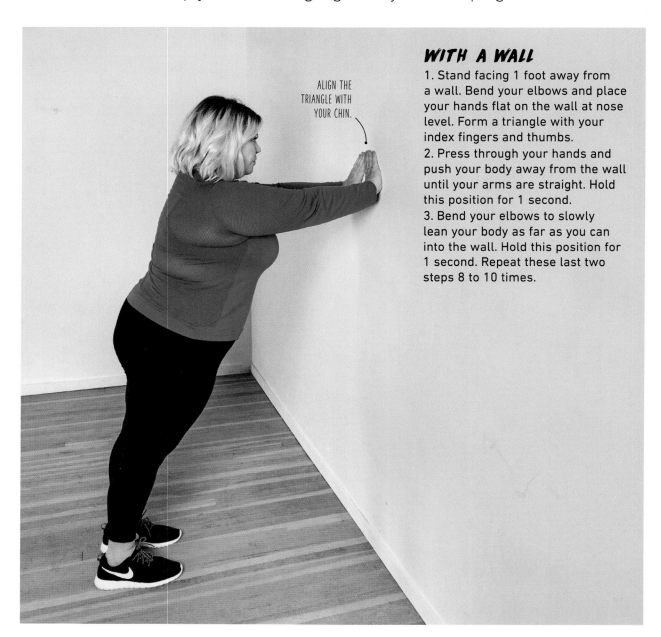

ALIGN THE
TRIANGLE WITH
YOUR CHIN.

WITH A WALL

1. Stand facing 1 foot away from a wall. Bend your elbows and place your hands flat on the wall at nose level. Form a triangle with your index fingers and thumbs.
2. Press through your hands and push your body away from the wall until your arms are straight. Hold this position for 1 second.
3. Bend your elbows to slowly lean your body as far as you can into the wall. Hold this position for 1 second. Repeat these last two steps 8 to 10 times.

KNEES ON THE FLOOR

1. Place your hands, knees, and the tops of your feet flat on the floor. Bend your elbows. Form a triangle with your index fingers and thumbs.

2. Push through your hands and lift your body off the floor until your arms are straight. Hold this position for 1 second.

3. Bend your elbows to slowly lower your body as far as you can. Hold this position for 1 second. Repeat these last two steps 8 to 10 times.

KEEP YOUR SHOULDERS DOWN.

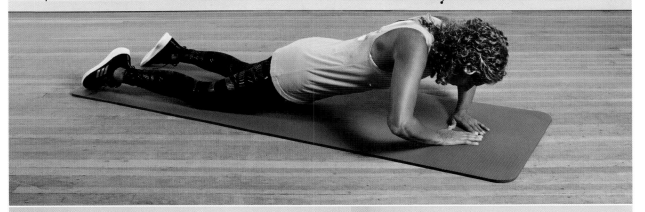

WITH A CHAIR

1. Place the back of a chair against a wall. Place your hands on the seat of the chair to form a triangle with your index fingers and thumbs. Extend your legs backward at a comfortable angle.

2. Push through your hands and lift your body off the chair until your arms are straight. Hold this position for 1 second.

3. Bend your elbows to slowly lower your body as far as you can toward the chair. Hold this position for 1 second. Repeat these last two steps 8 to 10 times.

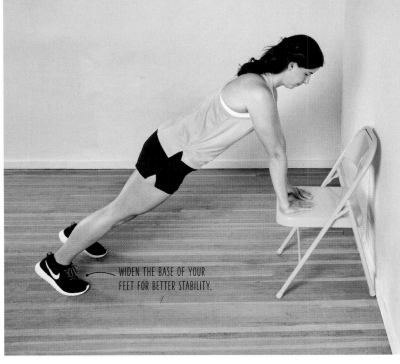

WIDEN THE BASE OF YOUR FEET FOR BETTER STABILITY.

PULLOVER

This exercise isolates your latissimus dorsi (lats), which are the large muscles that run down the sides of your back under your armpits. Strengthening these muscles can help you with lifting, rotating your arms, and pulling objects toward you.

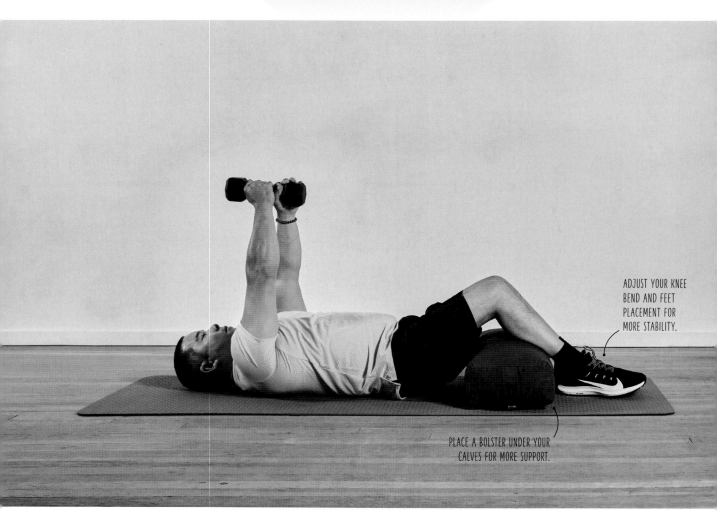

ADJUST YOUR KNEE BEND AND FEET PLACEMENT FOR MORE STABILITY.

PLACE A BOLSTER UNDER YOUR CALVES FOR MORE SUPPORT.

1 Lie on your back on the floor. Bend your knees at 45-degree angles and place your feet flat on the floor. Hold one weight in your hands and extend your arms toward the ceiling.

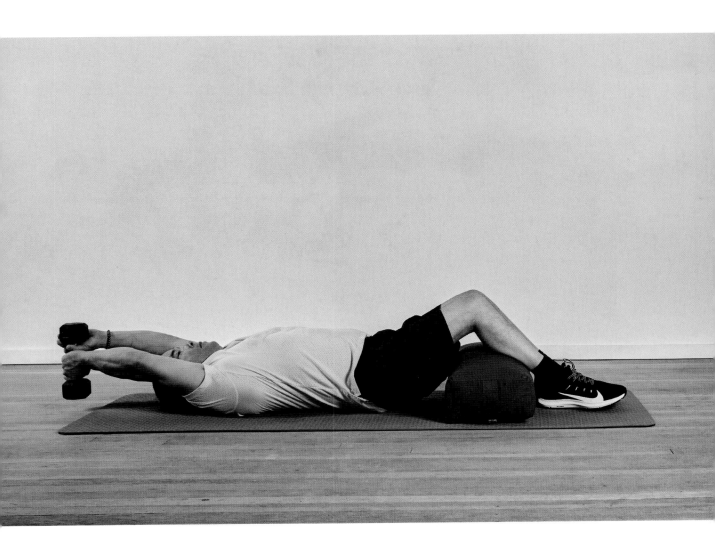

2 Slowly extend your arms over your head and lower the weight as close to the floor as possible. Pause, then extend your arms toward the ceiling. Repeat this step 8 to 10 times.

// PULLOVER //
VARIATIONS

If you find it challenging to get down on the floor,
try one of these modifications to do this exercise in another way.

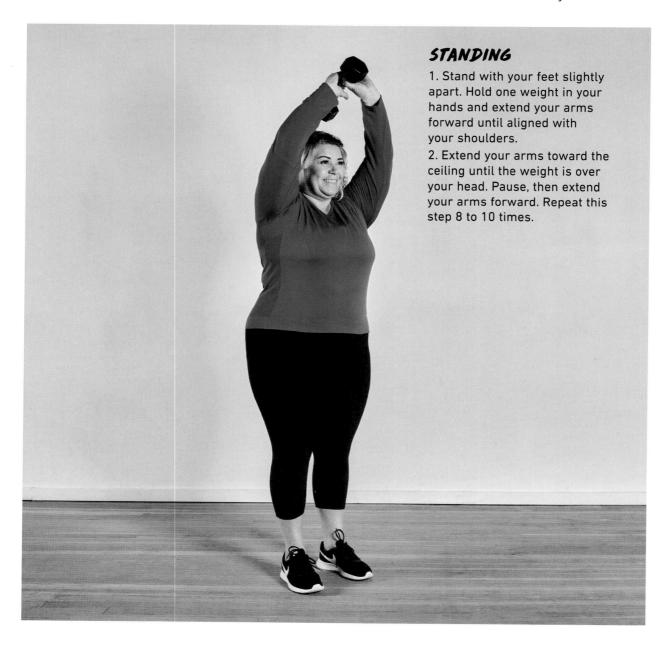

STANDING

1. Stand with your feet slightly apart. Hold one weight in your hands and extend your arms forward until aligned with your shoulders.

2. Extend your arms toward the ceiling until the weight is over your head. Pause, then extend your arms forward. Repeat this step 8 to 10 times.

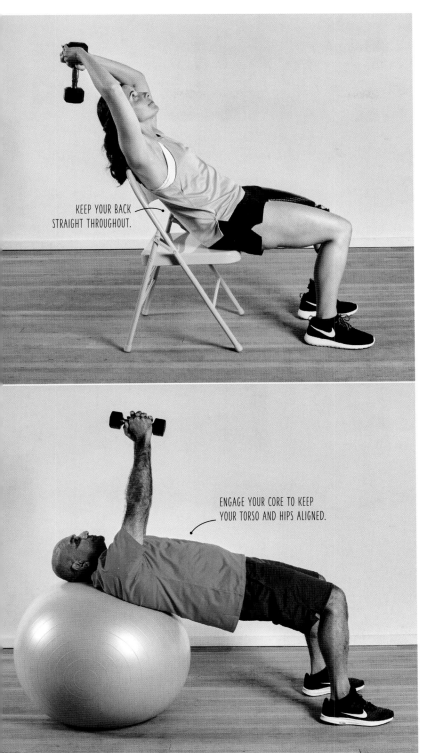

KEEP YOUR BACK STRAIGHT THROUGHOUT.

ENGAGE YOUR CORE TO KEEP YOUR TORSO AND HIPS ALIGNED.

SEATED

1. Sit on the edge of the seat of a chair and place your feet flat on the floor. Hold one weight in your hands and extend your arms toward the ceiling.

2. Lean backward until your upper back and shoulders are supported by the back of the chair. Slowly lower the weight behind your head. Pause, then extend your arms toward the ceiling. Repeat this step 8 to 10 times.

ON A STABILITY BALL

1. Lie on your back on a stability ball and position your mid- to upper back as the anchor on the ball. Place your feet flat on the floor under your knees. Hold one weight in your hands and extend your arms toward the ceiling. (You can place your feet or toes against a wall for more stability.)

2. Raise your hips until they align with your torso. Extend your arms over your head and slowly lower the weight behind your head. Pause, then extend your arms toward the ceiling. Repeat this step 8 to 10 times.

TRICEPS DIP

The triceps dip is a challenging but muscle-isolating exercise. It's challenging because the mechanics of the movements essentially put all your body weight in a smaller muscle group at the back of your arms while you dip.

1 Place the back of a chair against a wall. Stand facing away from the seat of the chair and relax your arms at your sides.

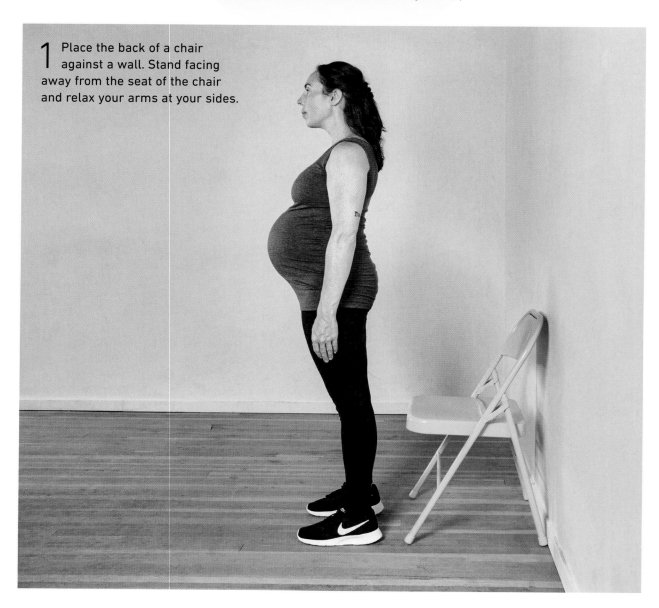

2 Bend your knees and lower yourself toward the seat of the chair. Place your hands on the sides of the chair and step your feet slightly forward.

KEEP YOUR FEET FLAT ON THE FLOOR.

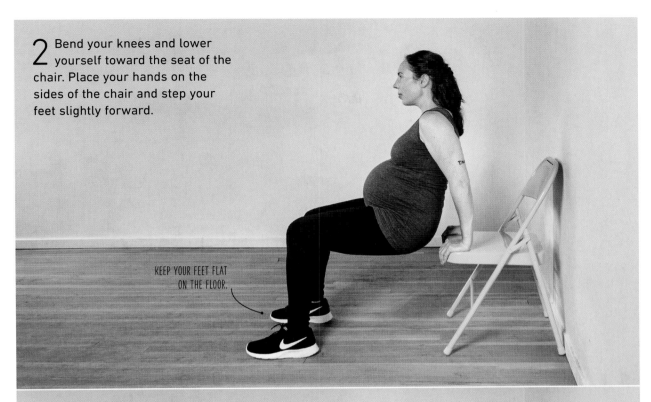

3 Bend your elbows to lower yourself toward the floor. Pause for 1 second, then straighten your arms. Repeat this step 8 to 10 times.

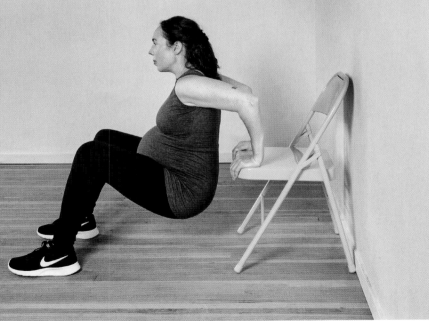

// TRICEPS DIP //

VARIATIONS

Try these seated, wall, and feet-stacking modifications
to help you work toward the main exercise.

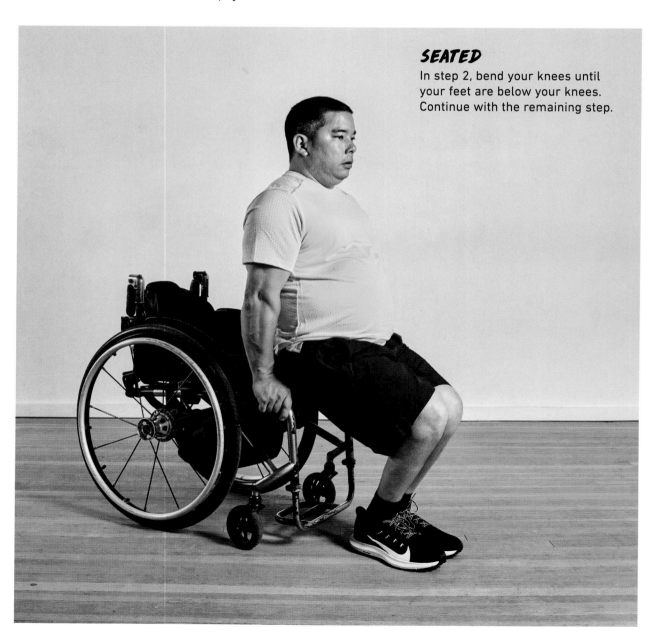

SEATED

In step 2, bend your knees until
your feet are below your knees.
Continue with the remaining step.

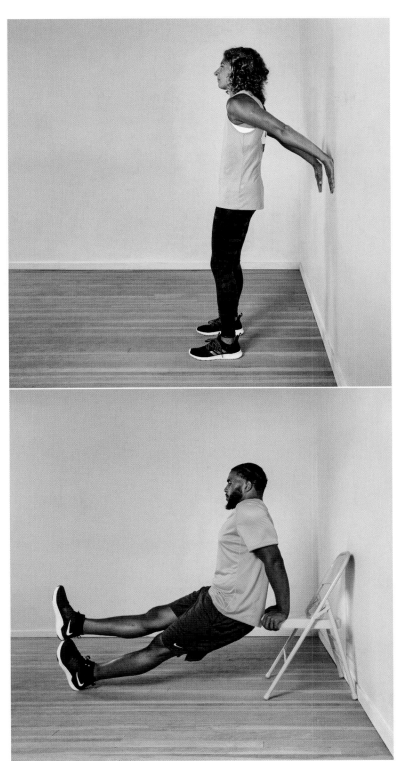

WITH A WALL

1. Stand with your back flat against a wall and place your hands flat against the wall just above your hips.

2. Step about 1 to 2 feet away from the wall and slightly bend your knees. Keep your elbows bent.

3. Push through your hands to lift your body off the wall until your arms are straight, then pause.

4. Bend your elbows to lower yourself toward the wall, then pause. Repeat these last two steps 8 to 10 times.

WITH A CHAIR

1. Stand facing away from the seat of a chair placed against a wall and relax your arms at your sides.

2. Bend your knees and lower yourself toward the floor.

3. Bend your elbows at 45-degree angles and place your hands on the sides of the chair. Extend your legs forward and place your right foot on top of your left foot (heel to toe). Pause, then straighten your arms. Repeat this step 8 to 10 times.

SIMI ATHWAL

I'm compassionate, hardworking, shy, and reserved at times, but I have a disciplined and goal-oriented attitude toward life. I have a competitive spirit in me that brings me great joy when I meet and surpass a challenge.

Ever since my parents and I emigrated from India to North America, being physically active has always been a part of my upbringing. From competing nationally in table tennis events as a child, push-up and chin-up contests, playing tennis and squash, running in local and international races and marathons, and, most recently, playing senior ladies doubles in tennis, I never sit still for long. Staying active and eating well really hit home for me when I lost my mom to cancer at such an early age as well as several close friends.

I credit my weight training during my teenage years with giving me the physical confidence and mental determination to overcome any challenges I faced as I entered adulthood. And to this day, I rely on my work with weights to keep me strong and grounded in body and mind.

I loved long-distance running for the stability it provided to my mind as I battled through a difficult marriage breakup. Cross-training with yoga and weight training has kept me injury-free all these years, and at 58 years old, I recently suffered my first major injury while playing in a local tennis tournament. Although I completely tore my ACL and partially tore my MCL, I was back on the tennis court in 8 weeks. My recovery surprised my doctor and physiotherapist and was highly likely a result of my overall fitness level.

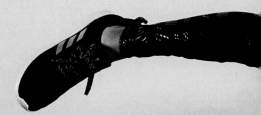

I raised my three boys—now also very active young adults—to keep moving and have fun in team sports like soccer, hockey, and, of course, tennis. I've prided myself in being a good role model for them and making fitness a key factor in maintaining joy and purpose in life. Needless to say, they're as competitive as me.

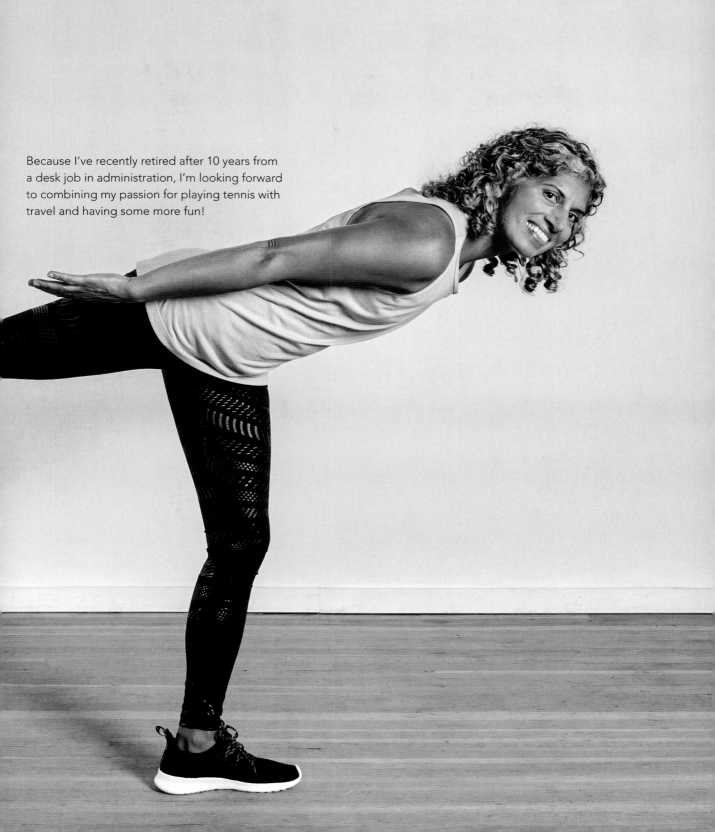

Because I've recently retired after 10 years from a desk job in administration, I'm looking forward to combining my passion for playing tennis with travel and having some more fun!

WOOD CHOP

These actions use the oblique plane of movement,
which involves rotation and diagonal motions. Plus, this exercise
uses all the planes of motion to keep the body tuned in to
a variety of movements, helping keep the brain alert.

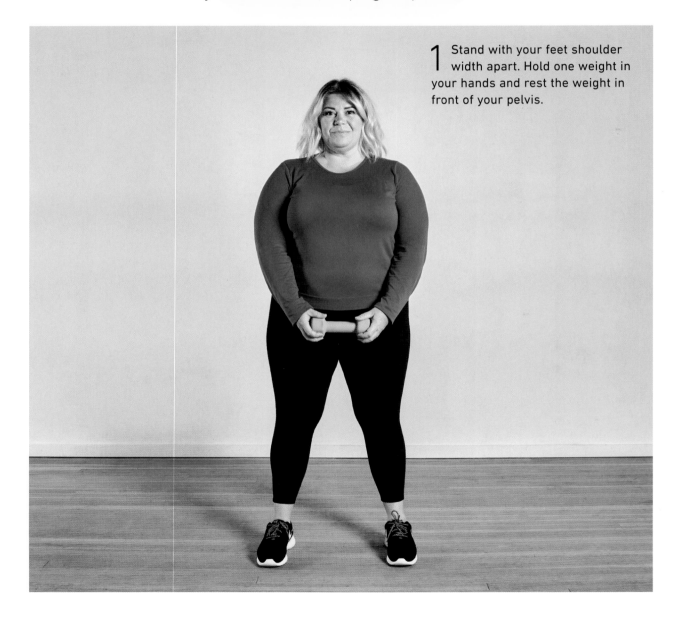

1 Stand with your feet shoulder width apart. Hold one weight in your hands and rest the weight in front of your pelvis.

2 Bend your knees to slowly lower your hips backward into a squat. Rotate your torso to your right and reach the weight toward the outside of your right leg.

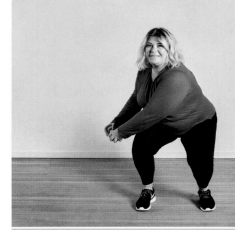

3 Begin to return to standing. Turn your right heel toward your right side and reach the weight toward your left shoulder. Pause, then return the weight to your right leg. Repeat this step 8 to 10 times.

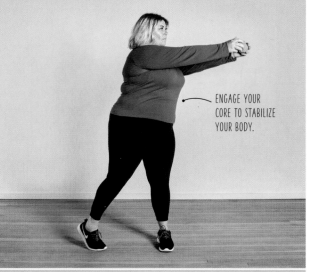

ENGAGE YOUR CORE TO STABILIZE YOUR BODY.

4 Bend your knees to slowly lower your hips backward into a squat. Rotate your torso to your left and reach the weight toward the outside of your left leg.

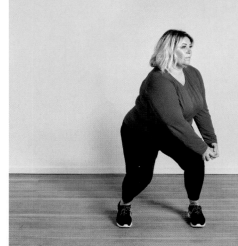

5 Begin to return to standing. Turn your left heel toward your left side and reach the weight toward your right shoulder. Pause, then return the weight to your left leg. Repeat this step 8 to 10 times.

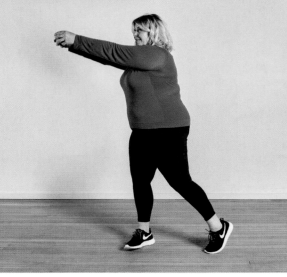

// WOOD CHOP //
VARIATIONS

If squatting isn't for you, try the standing version without weights or use a chair or a stability ball.

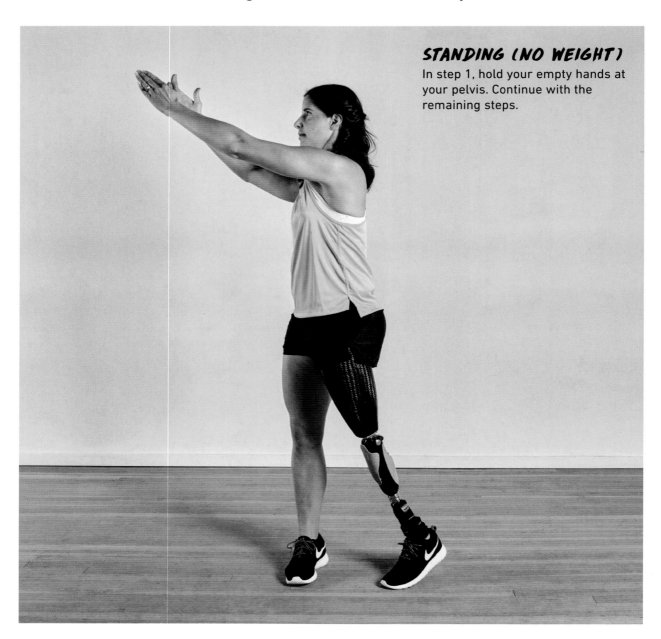

STANDING (NO WEIGHT)

In step 1, hold your empty hands at your pelvis. Continue with the remaining steps.

ON A STABILITY BALL

1. Sit on a stability ball and place your feet flat on the floor. Hold one weight in your hands and relax your arms at your right hip.
2. Raise the weight from your right hip across your body to your left shoulder. Pause, then lower the weight to your right hip. Repeat this step 8 to 10 times and lower the weight to your left hip after the last rep.
3. Raise the weight from your left hip across your body to your right shoulder. Pause, then lower the weight to your left hip. Repeat this step 8 to 10 times.

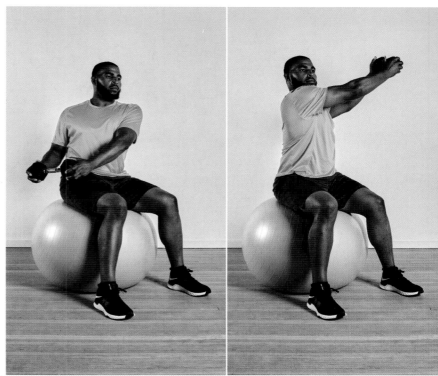

SEATED

1. Sit in a chair and place your feet flat on the floor. Hold one weight in your hands and relax your arms at your right hip.
2. Raise the weight from your right hip across your body to your left shoulder. Pause, then lower the weight to your right hip. Repeat this step 8 to 10 times and lower the weight to your left hip after the last rep.
3. Raise the weight from your left hip across your body to your right shoulder. Pause, then lower the weight to your left hip. Repeat this step 8 to 10 times.

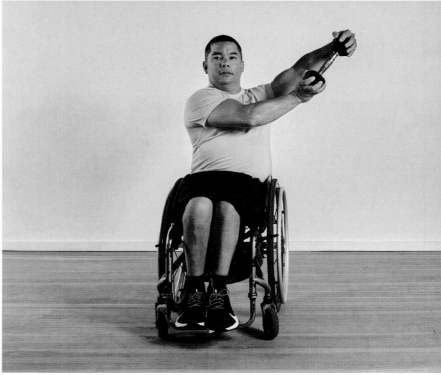

V-SIT OBLIQUE ROTATION

Oblique rotations target your middle abdominals and obliques—the muscles at the sides of your abs. When you recline, you work these muscles. More depth to your incline makes the demand more intense. Plus, when you rotate, you work your obliques.

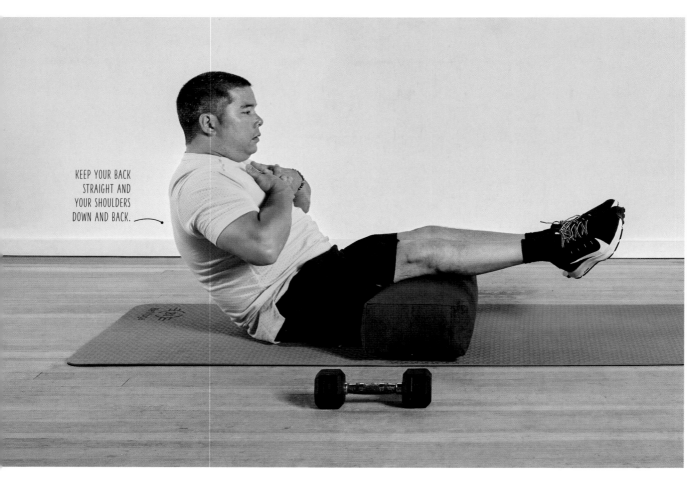

KEEP YOUR BACK STRAIGHT AND YOUR SHOULDERS DOWN AND BACK.

1 Sit on the floor and place a weight on the right side of your body. Place a bolster under your knees. Rest your hands at the center of your chest.

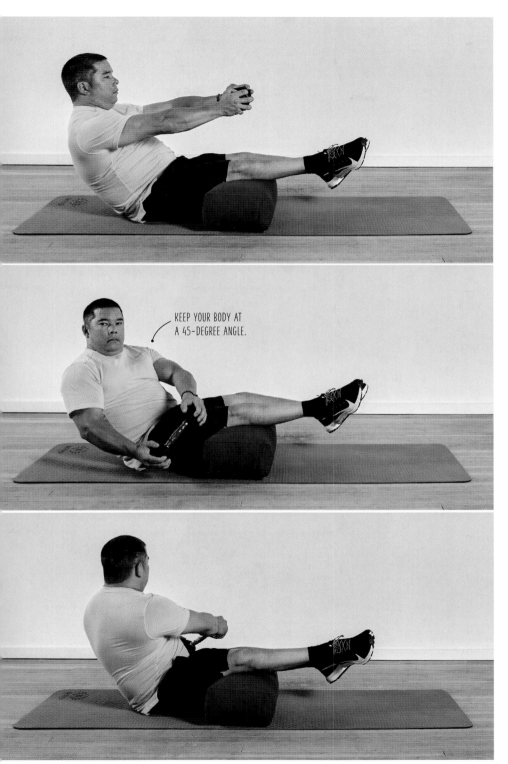

2 Grab the weight with your hands and extend your arms forward from your chest. Lean your torso back until you feel your core activated.

KEEP YOUR BODY AT A 45-DEGREE ANGLE.

3 Rotate your upper body to your right side and lower the weight to your right hip. Hold this position for 1 second.

4 Rotate your upper body to your left side and lower the weight to your left hip. Hold this position for 1 second. Repeat these last two steps 8 to 10 times per side.

// V-SIT OBLIQUE ROTATION //

VARIATIONS

You can do this exercise standing or you can challenge yourself more on the floor with either your feet anchored or unanchored.

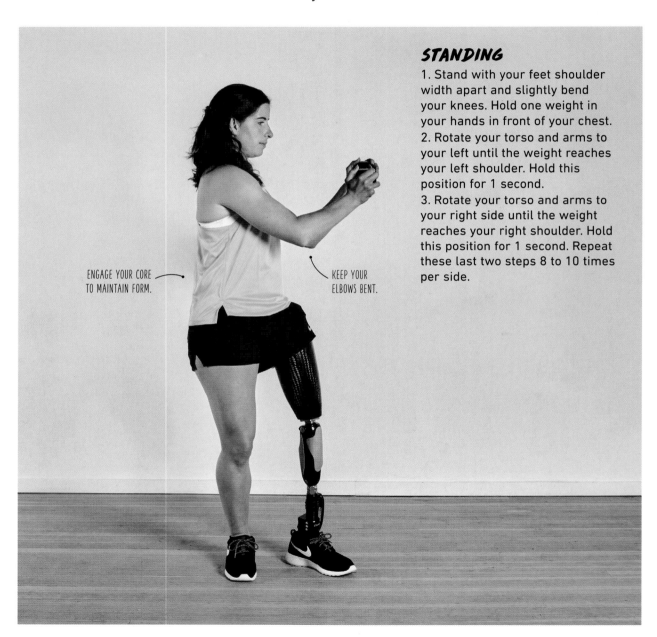

ENGAGE YOUR CORE
TO MAINTAIN FORM.

KEEP YOUR
ELBOWS BENT.

STANDING

1. Stand with your feet shoulder width apart and slightly bend your knees. Hold one weight in your hands in front of your chest.

2. Rotate your torso and arms to your left until the weight reaches your left shoulder. Hold this position for 1 second.

3. Rotate your torso and arms to your right side until the weight reaches your right shoulder. Hold this position for 1 second. Repeat these last two steps 8 to 10 times per side.

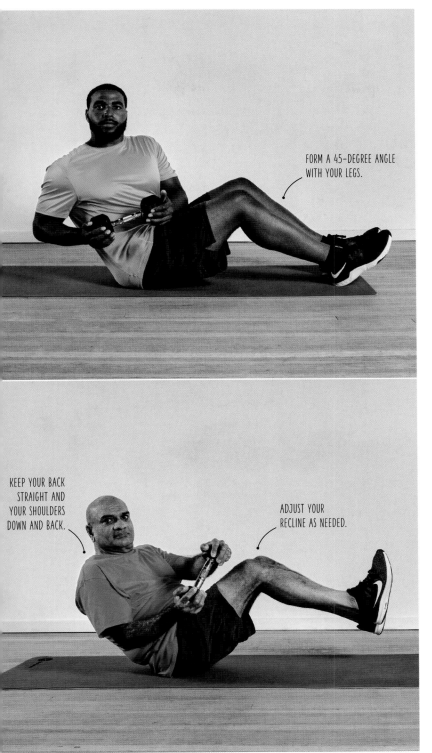

FORM A 45-DEGREE ANGLE WITH YOUR LEGS.

KEEP YOUR BACK STRAIGHT AND YOUR SHOULDERS DOWN AND BACK.

ADJUST YOUR RECLINE AS NEEDED.

FEET ON THE FLOOR

In step 1, bend your knees and press your heels into the floor rather than use a bolster. Continue with the remaining steps.

FEET ELEVATED

1. Sit on the floor and place a weight on the right side of your body. Lift your feet off the floor and bend your knees to form a 45-degree angle with your legs.

2. Grab the weight with your hands and extend your arms forward. Lean your torso backward to form a 45-degree angle with your body.

3. Rotate your torso and arms to your right side until the weight reaches your right hip. Hold this position for 1 second.

4. Rotate your torso and arms to your left side until the weight reaches your left hip. Hold this position for 1 second. Repeat these last two steps 8 to 10 times per side.

UPRIGHT PULL

This shoulder exercise focuses on your anterior and medial deltoids (the front and middle shoulder heads). Strengthening your deltoids can help you prevent shoulder injuries. Thus, for shoulder health, perform these upright pulls with lighter weights.

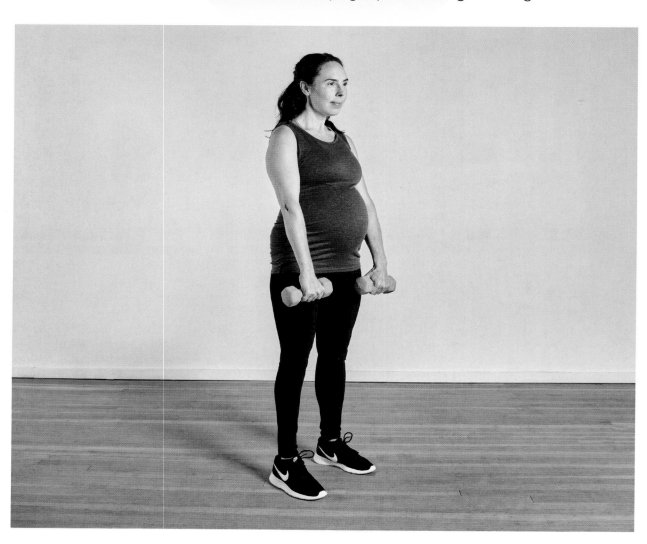

1 Stand with your feet shoulder width apart. Hold a weight in each hand and rest the weights on your thighs.

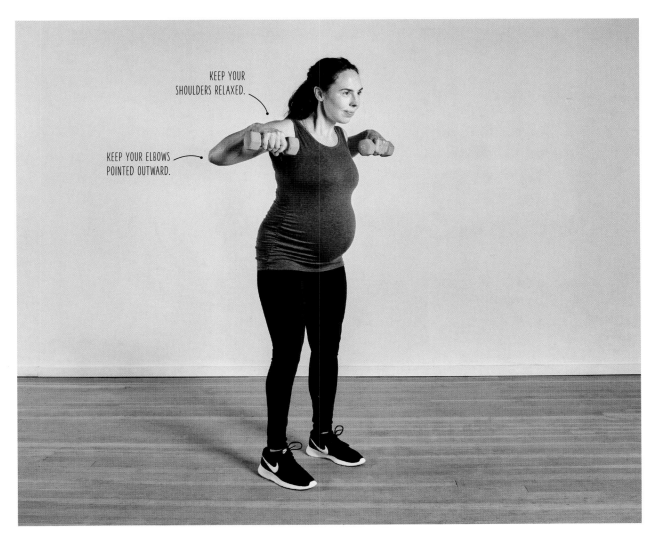

KEEP YOUR
SHOULDERS RELAXED.

KEEP YOUR ELBOWS
POINTED OUTWARD.

2 Lift your arms until the weights align with your shoulders. Pause, then lower your arms to your thighs. Repeat this step 8 to 10 times.

// UPRIGHT PULL //
VARIATIONS

Try the seated option if you have trouble standing
or try the split stance or shoulder roll to add more challenge.

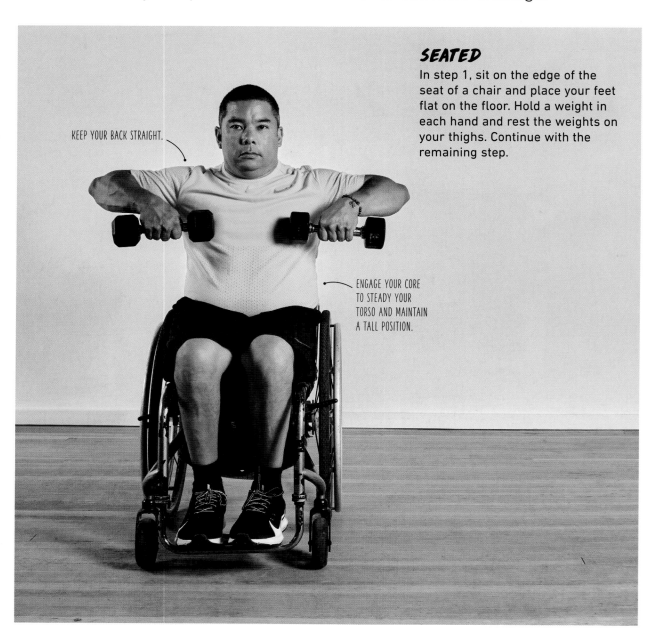

KEEP YOUR BACK STRAIGHT.

SEATED

In step 1, sit on the edge of the seat of a chair and place your feet flat on the floor. Hold a weight in each hand and rest the weights on your thighs. Continue with the remaining step.

ENGAGE YOUR CORE
TO STEADY YOUR
TORSO AND MAINTAIN
A TALL POSITION.

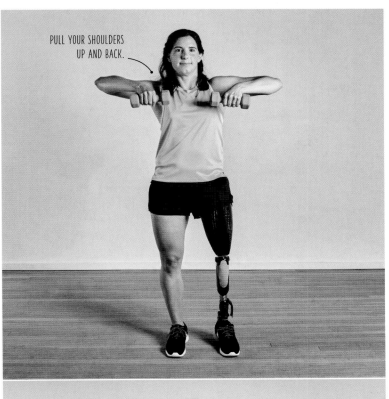

PULL YOUR SHOULDERS UP AND BACK.

WITH LESS INTENSITY

In step 2, as the weights reach your shoulders, round your shoulders up and back. Continue with the remainder of the step.

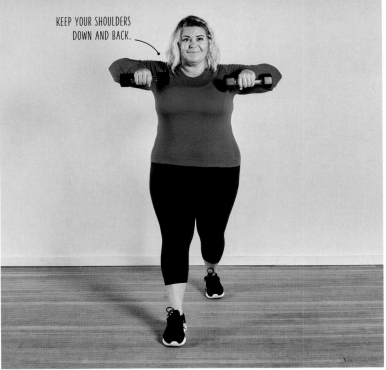

KEEP YOUR SHOULDERS DOWN AND BACK.

WITH A SPLIT STANCE

1. Stand with your feet shoulder width apart and slightly bend your knees. Hold a weight in each hand and relax your arms at your sides.
2. Step your right foot forward, exaggerating your natural stride by about 2 feet, to form a triangle with your body.
3. Lift your arms until the weights align with your shoulders. Pause, then lower the weights to your hips. Repeat this step 8 to 10 times. Repeat these steps with your left foot stepped forward.

BENT-OVER ROW

This exercise isolates and works your upper back muscles, specifically the rhomboids, lats, and trapezius. For this to be most effective, you need to bend your body to at least a 45-degree angle to keep this as a back exercise.

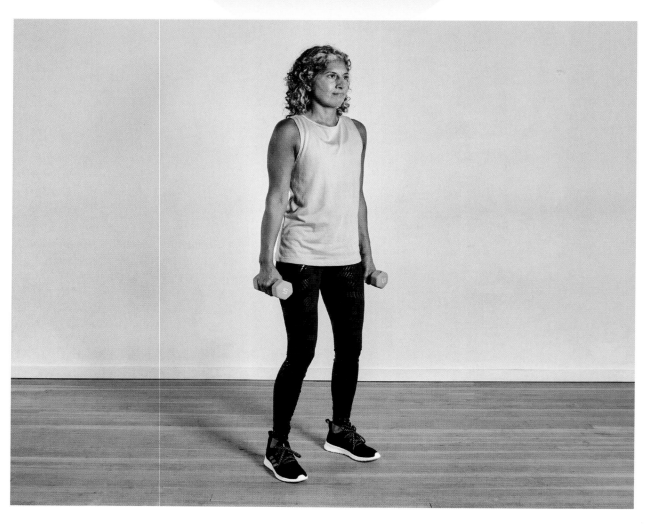

1 Stand with your feet shoulder width apart and slightly bend your knees. Hold a weight in each hand and relax your arms at your sides.

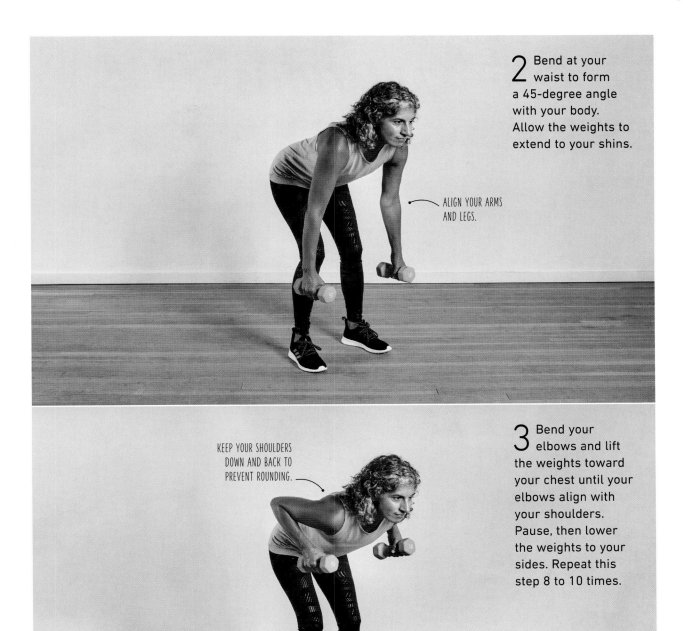

2 Bend at your waist to form a 45-degree angle with your body. Allow the weights to extend to your shins.

ALIGN YOUR ARMS AND LEGS.

KEEP YOUR SHOULDERS DOWN AND BACK TO PREVENT ROUNDING.

3 Bend your elbows and lift the weights toward your chest until your elbows align with your shoulders. Pause, then lower the weights to your sides. Repeat this step 8 to 10 times.

// BENT-OVER ROW //

VARIATIONS

These variations offer ways to make this exercise
more challenging through balance or easier with chair options.

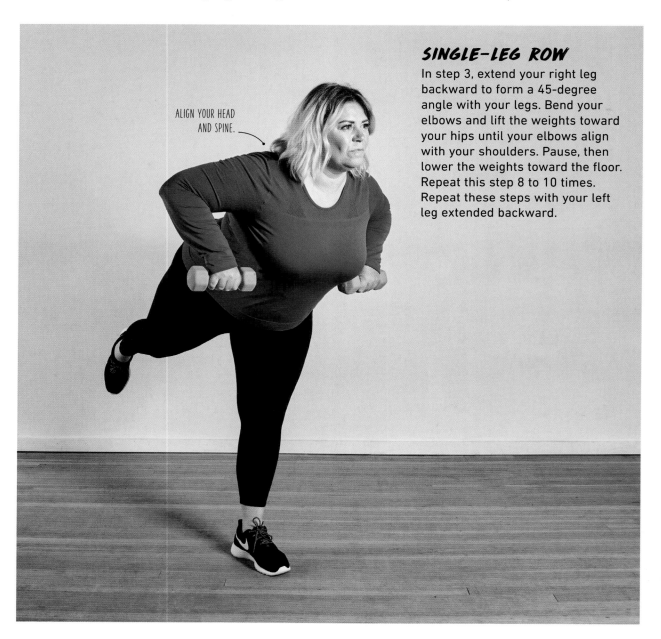

ALIGN YOUR HEAD
AND SPINE.

SINGLE-LEG ROW

In step 3, extend your right leg
backward to form a 45-degree
angle with your legs. Bend your
elbows and lift the weights toward
your hips until your elbows align
with your shoulders. Pause, then
lower the weights toward the floor.
Repeat this step 8 to 10 times.
Repeat these steps with your left
leg extended backward.

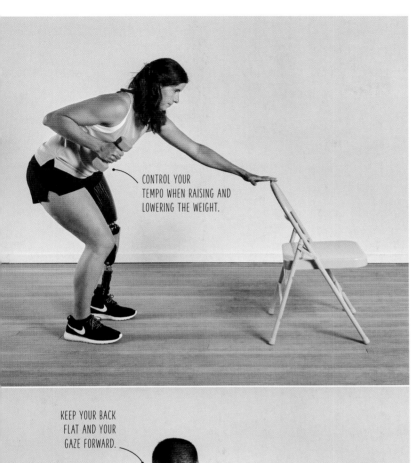

CONTROL YOUR TEMPO WHEN RAISING AND LOWERING THE WEIGHT.

WITH A CHAIR

1. Stand 1 to 2 feet behind a chair facing away from you. Hold a weight in your right hand and relax your right arm at your side. Place your left hand on the back of the chair.

2. Bend at your waist to form a 45-degree angle with your body.

3. Bend your right elbow and lift the weight toward the right side of your chest. Pause, then lower the weight to your side. Repeat this step 8 to 10 times. Repeat these steps with a weight in your left hand and your right hand on the back of the chair.

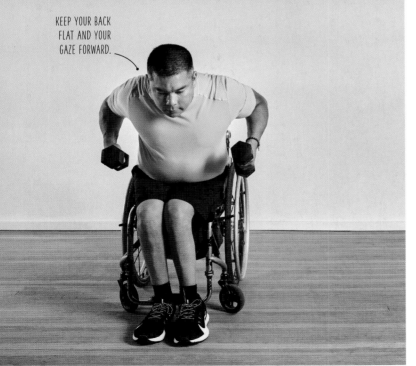

KEEP YOUR BACK FLAT AND YOUR GAZE FORWARD.

SEATED

1. Sit on the edge of the seat of a chair. Hold a weight in each hand and relax your arms at your sides.

2. Bend at your waist to form a 45-degree angle with your body.

3. Bend your elbows and lift the weights toward your hips. Pause, then lower the weights to your sides. Repeat this step 8 to 10 times.

SUPERHERO
(LOWER BACK EXTENSION)

Low back pain is often the result of weakness in your lower back.
So why would you want to do a lower back extension?
Because gently performing these steps can help you slowly
build strength in your lower back and reduce discomfort.

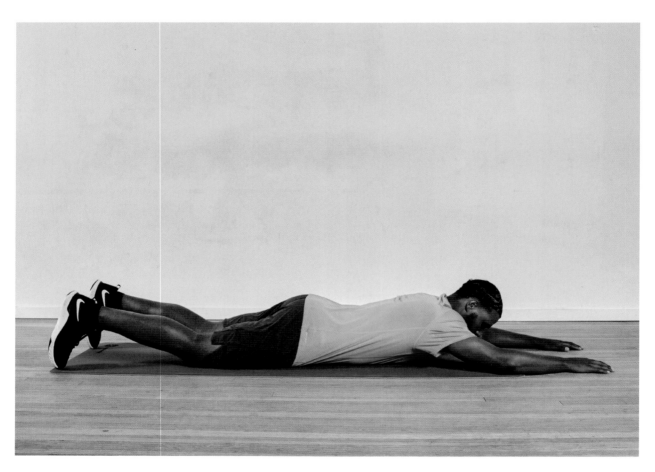

1 Lie on your stomach on the floor. Extend your
arms forward and extend your legs backward.

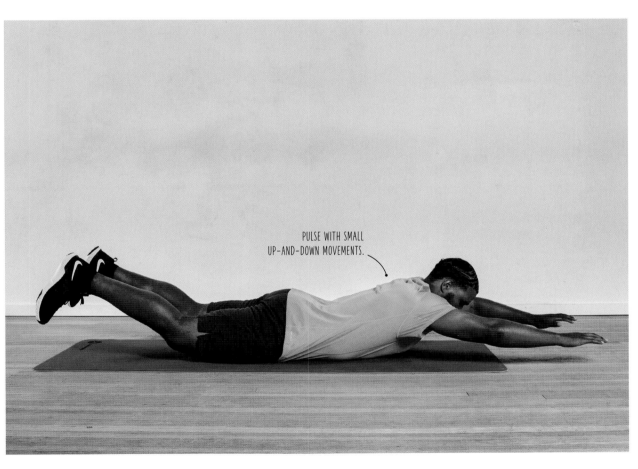

PULSE WITH SMALL
UP-AND-DOWN MOVEMENTS.

2 Raise your arms, lower legs, and chest off
the floor. Hold this position for 2 to 3 seconds,
then lower your body to the floor. Repeat this step
8 to 10 times.

// SUPERHERO (LOWER BACK EXTENSION) //
VARIATIONS

Use a chair to stay off the floor or use a stability ball to intensify core activation. Try the tabletop modification for a little variety.

WITH A CHAIR

1. Face the seat of a chair toward a wall. Stand behind the chair with your feet shoulder width apart. Place your right hand on the back of the chair and relax your left arm at your side.

2. Bend at your waist to form a 45-degree angle with your body. Extend your left arm toward the wall until parallel with the floor and extend your right leg backward. Hold this position for 2 to 3 seconds, then lower your left arm to your side and your right leg to the floor.

3. Extend your right arm toward the wall until parallel with the floor and extend your left leg backward. Hold this position for 2 to 3 seconds, then lower your right arm to your side and your left leg to the floor. Repeat these last two steps 8 to 10 times.

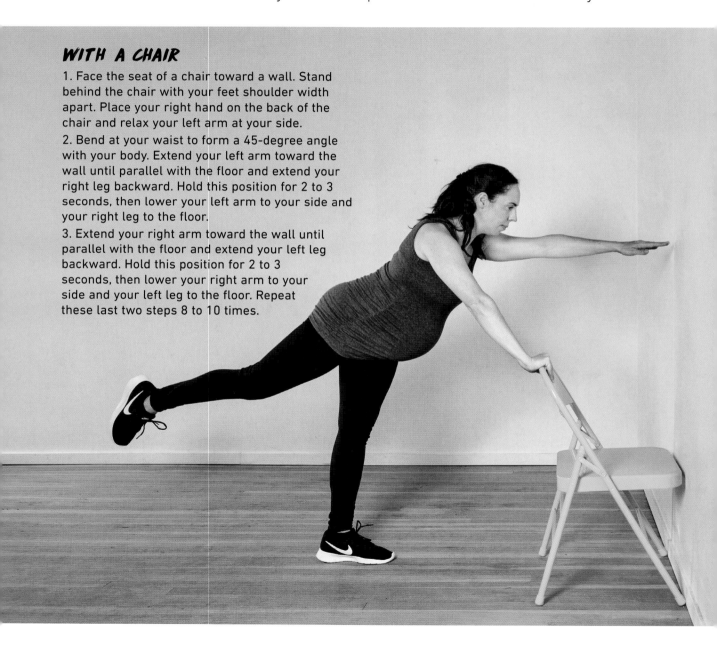

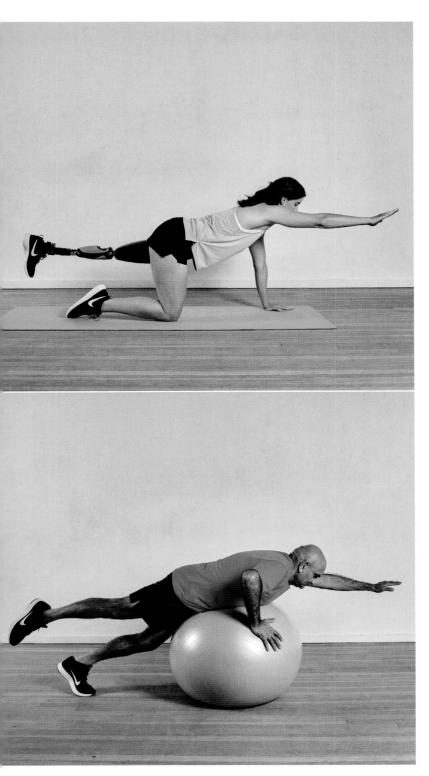

ON THE FLOOR

1. Place your hands, knees, and the tops of your feet flat on the floor.

2. Slowly extend your right arm forward and extend your left leg backward. Hold this position for 2 to 3 seconds, then lower your right arm and left leg to the floor.

3. Slowly extend your left arm forward and extend your right leg backward. Hold this position for 2 to 3 seconds, then lower your left arm and right leg to the floor. Repeat these last two steps 8 to 10 times.

ON A STABILITY BALL

1. Lie on your stomach on a stability ball. Place your hands flat on the floor or on the ball to stabilize your body. Extend your legs backward.

2. Slowly extend your left arm forward and extend your right leg backward. Hold this position for 2 to 3 seconds, then return your left arm and right leg to their starting positions.

3. Slowly extend your right arm forward and extend your left leg backward. Hold this position for 2 to 3 seconds, then return your right arm and left leg to their starting positions. Repeat these last two steps 8 to 10 times.

UPRIGHT PLANK

Upright planks use the strength of your body to elevate and hold your body weight. This forces the core to engage and stabilize the body. This plank is a good place to start for a highly effective exercise for building core strength.

1 Place your hands, knees, and the tops of your feet flat on the floor. (You can also place a bolster under your feet for more support.)

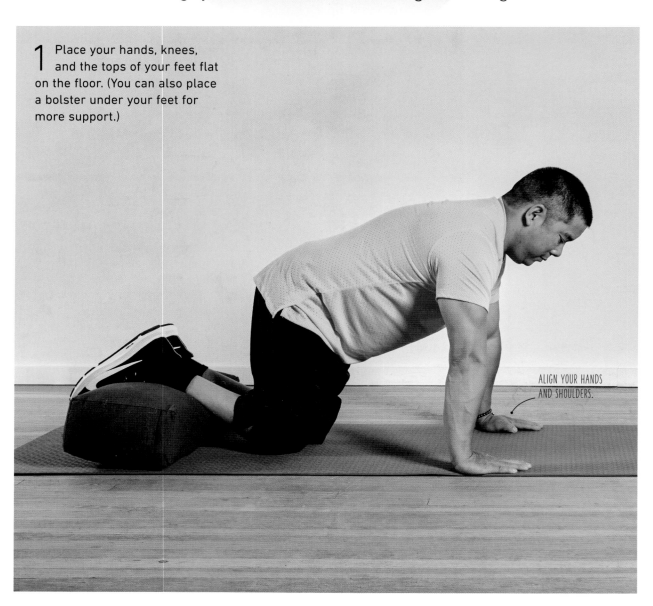

ALIGN YOUR HANDS AND SHOULDERS.

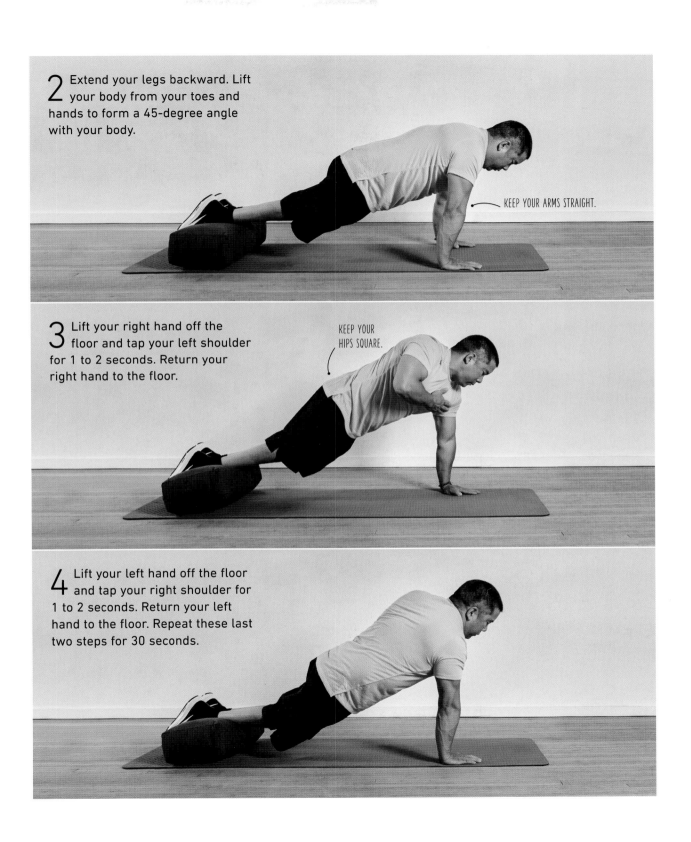

2 Extend your legs backward. Lift your body from your toes and hands to form a 45-degree angle with your body.

KEEP YOUR ARMS STRAIGHT.

3 Lift your right hand off the floor and tap your left shoulder for 1 to 2 seconds. Return your right hand to the floor.

KEEP YOUR HIPS SQUARE.

4 Lift your left hand off the floor and tap your right shoulder for 1 to 2 seconds. Return your left hand to the floor. Repeat these last two steps for 30 seconds.

// UPRIGHT PLANK //
VARIATIONS

Planking often needs to be done gradually. These options let you ease into a plank with elevated surfaces but without taps.

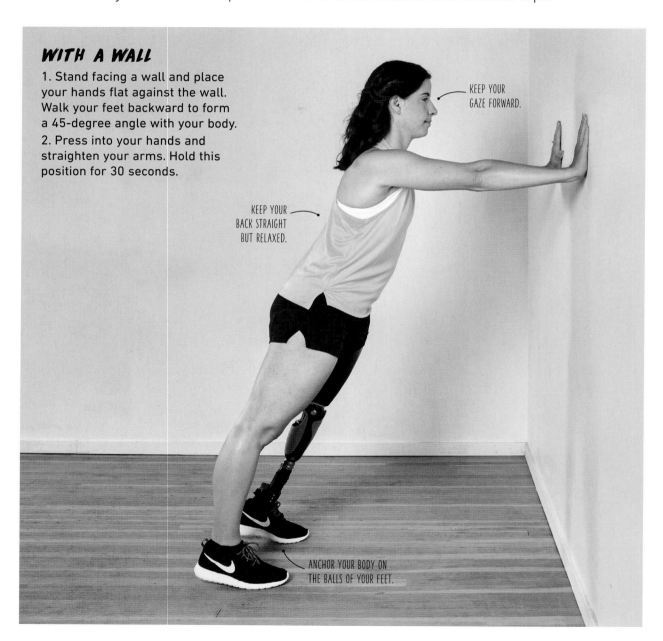

WITH A WALL

1. Stand facing a wall and place your hands flat against the wall. Walk your feet backward to form a 45-degree angle with your body.
2. Press into your hands and straighten your arms. Hold this position for 30 seconds.

KEEP YOUR GAZE FORWARD.

KEEP YOUR BACK STRAIGHT BUT RELAXED.

ANCHOR YOUR BODY ON THE BALLS OF YOUR FEET.

WITH A CHAIR

In step 1, place the back of a chair against a wall. Place your hands on the seat of the chair. After step 2, hold the plank position for 30 seconds instead of tapping.

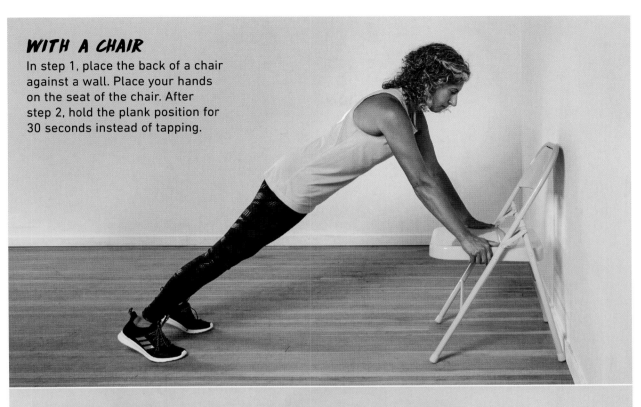

ON THE FLOOR

After step 2, hold the plank position for 30 seconds instead of tapping.

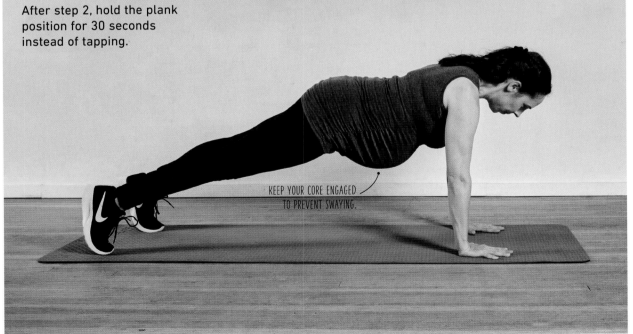

KEEP YOUR CORE ENGAGED TO PREVENT SWAYING.

LEG DROP

Performing an effective core exercise can engage your lower and middle abs (transverse and rectus abdominis). Leg drops typically have slow movements that isolate these abs, helping prevent back injuries as well as strengthening your posture.

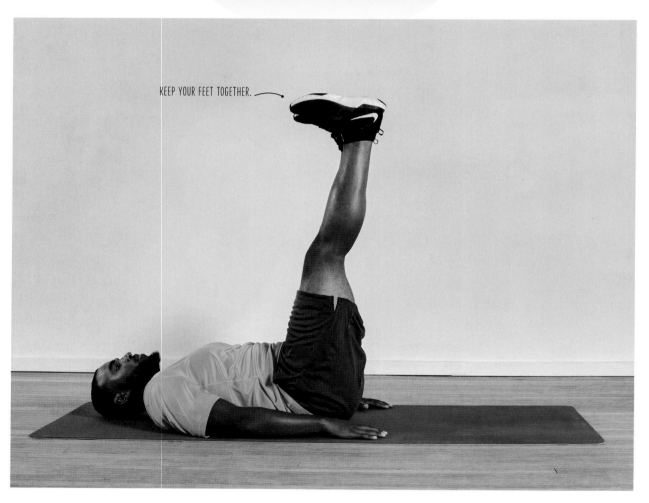

KEEP YOUR FEET TOGETHER.

1 Lie on your back on the floor and lift your legs to form a 90-degree angle with your body. Relax your arms at your sides.

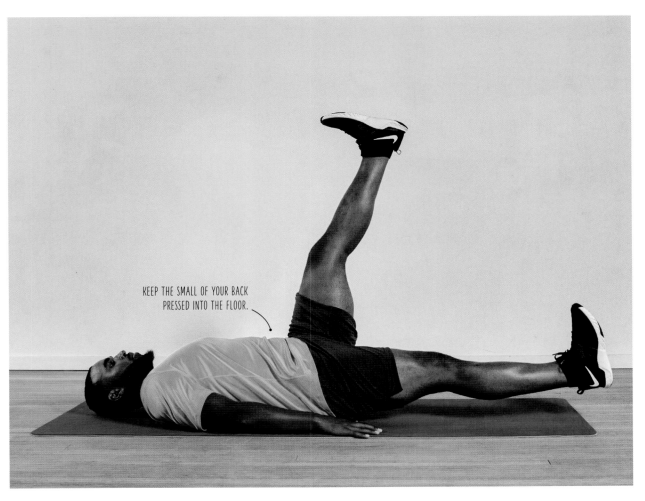

KEEP THE SMALL OF YOUR BACK
PRESSED INTO THE FLOOR.

2 Lower your right leg almost to the floor. Pause,
then return your right leg to its starting position.
Lower your left leg almost to the floor. Pause, then
return your left leg to its starting position. Repeat
this step 12 times.

// LEG DROP //

VARIATIONS

Use a chair to make this exercise more accessible
or you can increase the challenge with weights or lateral drops.

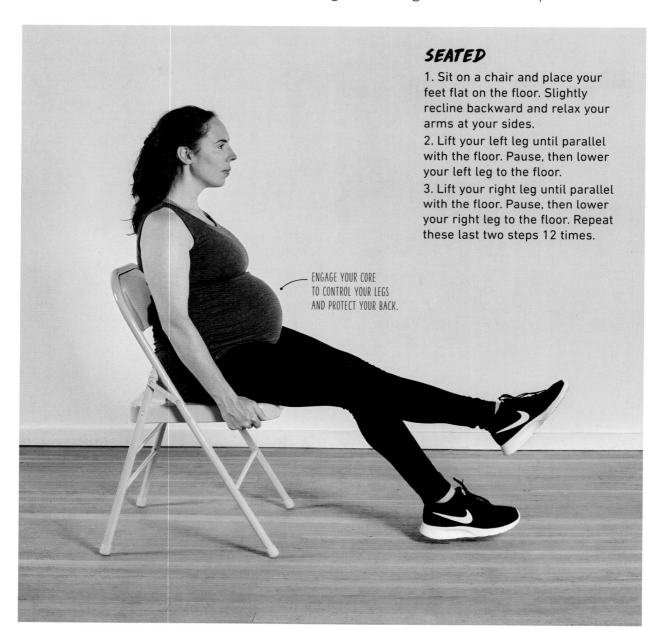

SEATED

1. Sit on a chair and place your feet flat on the floor. Slightly recline backward and relax your arms at your sides.

2. Lift your left leg until parallel with the floor. Pause, then lower your left leg to the floor.

3. Lift your right leg until parallel with the floor. Pause, then lower your right leg to the floor. Repeat these last two steps 12 times.

ENGAGE YOUR CORE TO CONTROL YOUR LEGS AND PROTECT YOUR BACK.

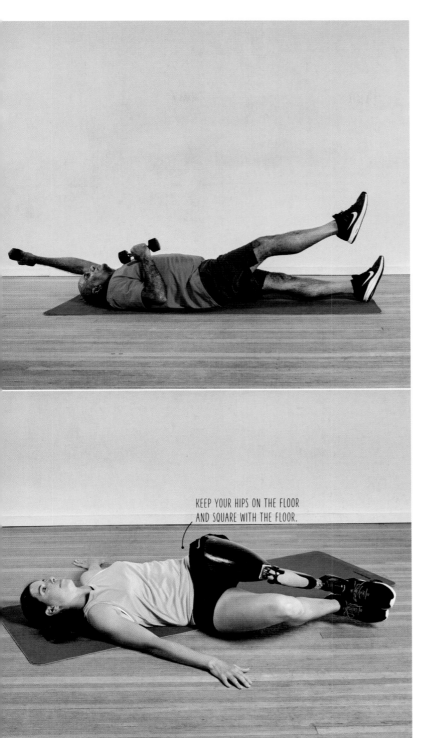

KEEP YOUR HIPS ON THE FLOOR AND SQUARE WITH THE FLOOR.

WITH WEIGHTS

1. Lie on your back on the floor. Hold a weight in each hand and rest the weights on your chest.

2. Raise your right leg off the floor and extend your left arm over your head. Pause, then lower your right leg to the floor and your left hand to your chest.

3. Raise your left leg off the floor and extend your right arm over your head. Pause, then lower your left leg to the floor and your right hand to your chest. Repeat these last two steps 8 to 12 times.

LATERAL MOVEMENT

1. Lie on your back on the floor and bend your knees to bring your legs toward your chest. Extend your arms to your sides and place your hands flat on the floor.

2. Slowly lower your legs toward your right side. Pause, then return your legs to center.

3. Slowly lower your legs toward your left side. Pause, then return your legs to center. Repeat these last two steps 12 times.

DEAD BUG

This is an excellent exercise for working your lower abdominals (transverse abdominals). Because these abs stabilize your pelvis and lower back when you move, strengthening this area is fundamental to your posture and sound movement mechanics.

1 Lie on your back on the floor and extend your arms toward the ceiling. Lift your legs and bend your knees to form a 90-degree angle with your legs.

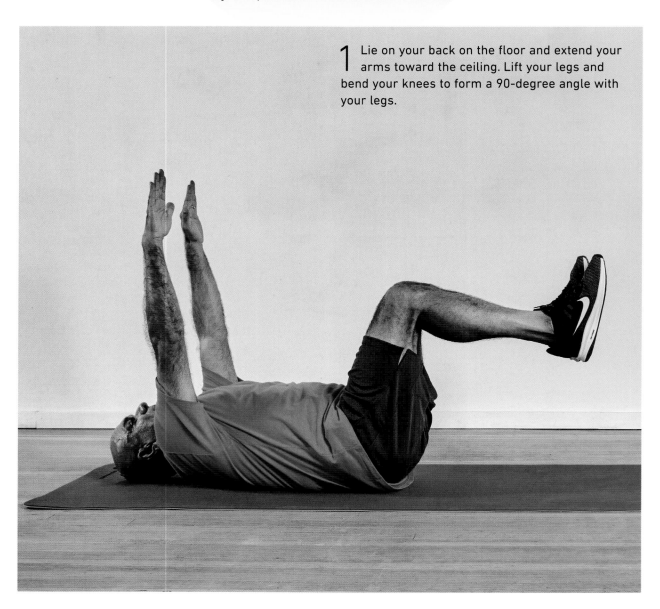

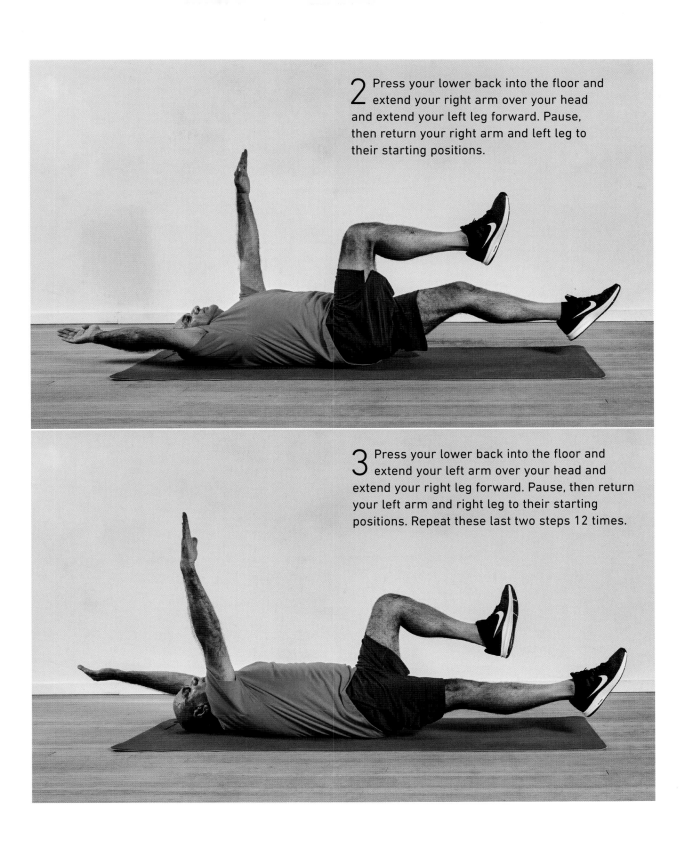

2 Press your lower back into the floor and extend your right arm over your head and extend your left leg forward. Pause, then return your right arm and left leg to their starting positions.

3 Press your lower back into the floor and extend your left arm over your head and extend your right leg forward. Pause, then return your left arm and right leg to their starting positions. Repeat these last two steps 12 times.

// DEAD BUG //

VARIATIONS

Everyone can be a dead bug with one of these options,
including performing the exercise while sitting or standing.

WITH A WALL

1. Stand with your back and heels flat against a wall. Relax your arms at your sides and against the wall.

2. Bend your left knee to slowly lift your left foot off the floor to form a 90-degree angle with your left leg. Extend your right arm forward until parallel with the floor. Pause, then return your left leg and right arm to the wall.

3. Bend your right knee to slowly lift your right foot off the floor to form a 90-degree angle with your right leg. Extend your left arm until parallel with the floor. Pause, then return your right leg and left arm to the wall. Repeat these last two steps 12 times.

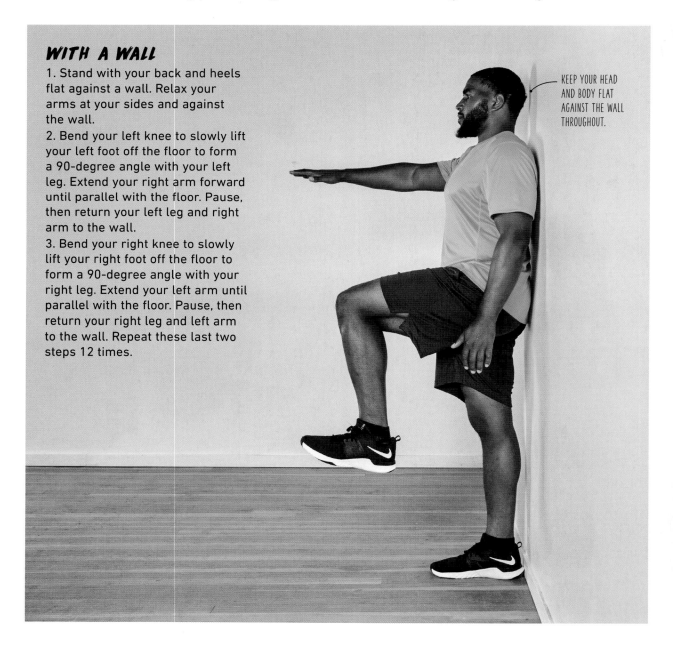

KEEP YOUR HEAD AND BODY FLAT AGAINST THE WALL THROUGHOUT.

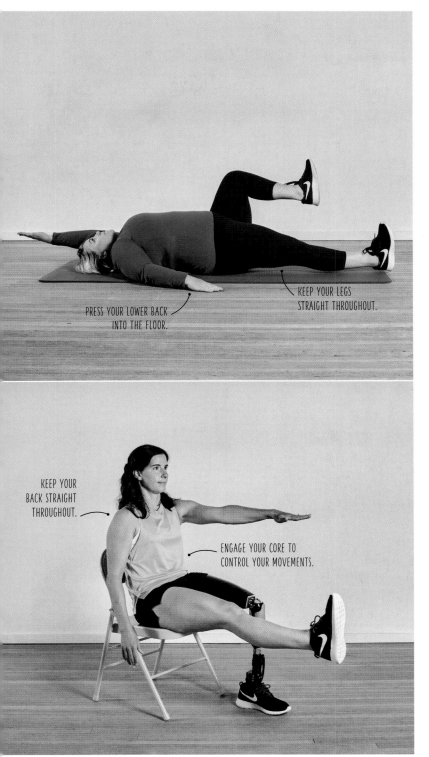

PRESS YOUR LOWER BACK INTO THE FLOOR.

KEEP YOUR LEGS STRAIGHT THROUGHOUT.

KEEP YOUR BACK STRAIGHT THROUGHOUT.

ENGAGE YOUR CORE TO CONTROL YOUR MOVEMENTS.

LEG ON THE FLOOR

1. Lie on your back on the floor and relax your arms at your sides. Bend your knees and lift your legs off the floor to form a 90-degree angle with your legs.

2. Extend your left arm over your head and lower your right leg until flat on the floor. Pause, then return your left arm to your left side and return your right leg to a 90-degree angle.

3. Extend your right arm over your head and lower your left leg until flat on the floor. Pause, then return your right arm to your right side and return your left leg to a 90-degree angle. Repeat these last two steps 12 times.

SEATED

1. Sit on the edge of the seat of a chair and place your feet flat on the floor. Relax your arms at your sides.

2. Lift your right leg and your left arm until parallel with the floor. Pause, then lower your right leg to the floor and your left arm to your side.

3. Lift your left leg and right arm until parallel with the floor. Pause, then lower your left leg to the floor and your right arm to your side. Repeat these last two steps 12 times.

BICEPS CURL

Biceps are an easy muscle to isolate with this exercise.
This specific curl is a great way to build strength in your arms,
helping you lift and carry with more ease for functional living.
Plus, who doesn't love the look of strong biceps?

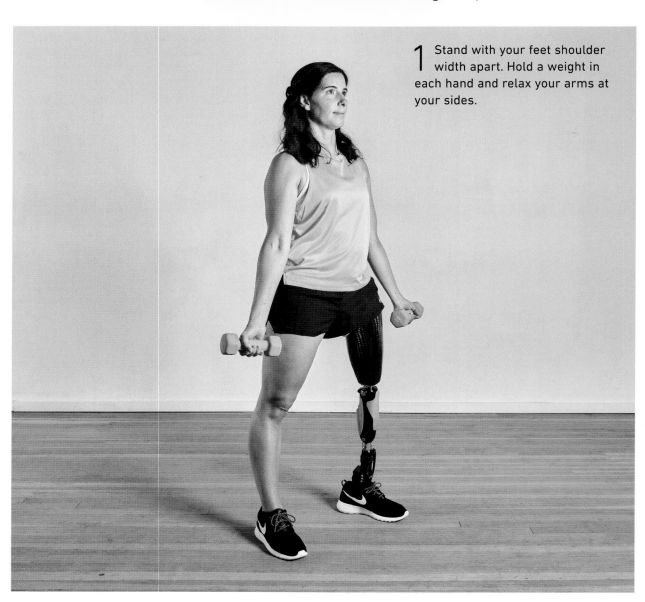

1 Stand with your feet shoulder width apart. Hold a weight in each hand and relax your arms at your sides.

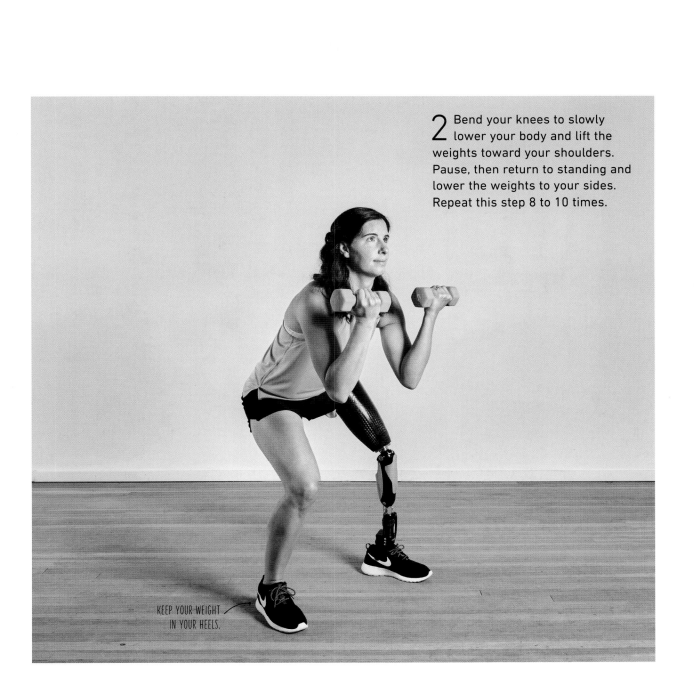

2 Bend your knees to slowly lower your body and lift the weights toward your shoulders. Pause, then return to standing and lower the weights to your sides. Repeat this step 8 to 10 times.

KEEP YOUR WEIGHT IN YOUR HEELS.

// BICEPS CURL //
VARIATIONS

These variations make this exercise less difficult by removing
the multi-joint movement and adding some seated options.

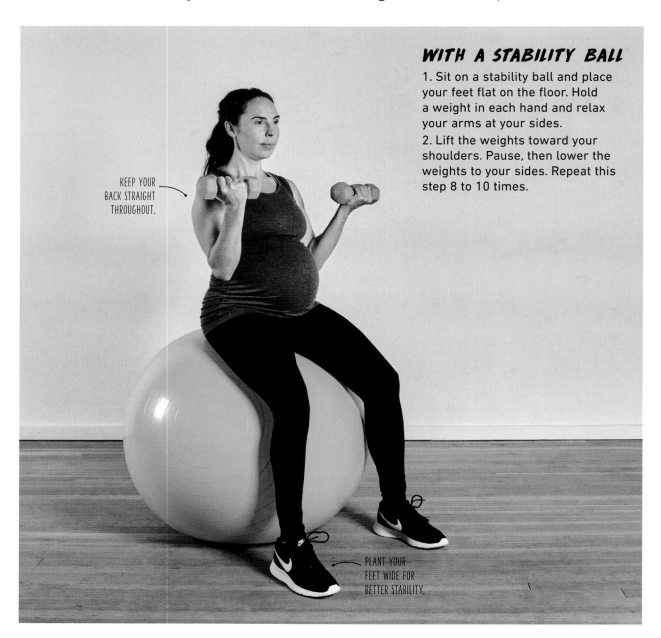

WITH A STABILITY BALL

1. Sit on a stability ball and place your feet flat on the floor. Hold a weight in each hand and relax your arms at your sides.
2. Lift the weights toward your shoulders. Pause, then lower the weights to your sides. Repeat this step 8 to 10 times.

KEEP YOUR BACK STRAIGHT THROUGHOUT.

PLANT YOUR FEET WIDE FOR BETTER STABILITY.

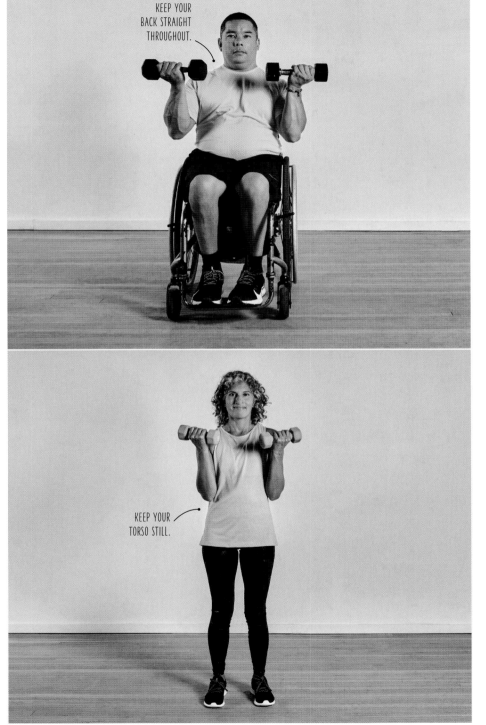

KEEP YOUR BACK STRAIGHT THROUGHOUT.

KEEP YOUR TORSO STILL.

SEATED

1. Sit in a chair and place your feet flat on the floor. Hold a weight in each hand and relax your arms at your sides.

2. Lift the weights toward your shoulders. Pause, then lower the weights to your sides. Repeat this step 8 to 10 times.

STANDING STRAIGHT

1. Stand with your feet shoulder width apart. Hold a weight in each hand and relax your arms at your sides.

2. Raise the weights to toward your shoulders. Pause, then lower the weights to your sides. Repeat this step 8 to 10 times.

SIDE PLANK

This exercise works the obliques in your core but also recruits your shoulders while you try to stabilize your body. Planking requires a good amount of balance because you're using just your feet and elbow to keep your body lifted.

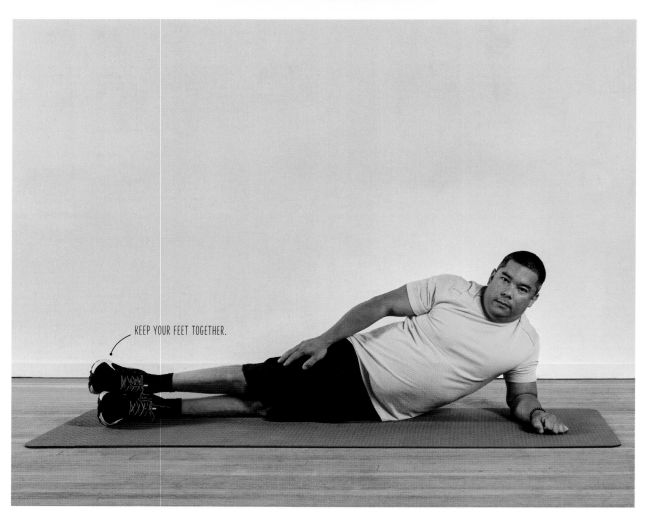

KEEP YOUR FEET TOGETHER.

1 Lie on your left side on the floor and place your left forearm flat on the floor below your left shoulder.

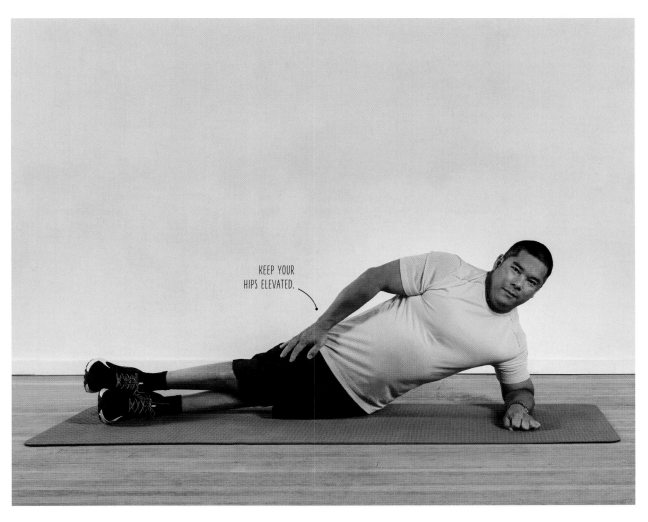

KEEP YOUR
HIPS ELEVATED.

2 Lift your hips until your body forms a straight
line from head to toe. Hold this position for
30 seconds, then lower your body to the floor.
Repeat these steps on your right side.

// SIDE PLANK //
VARIATIONS

These modifications make this a more accessible exercise
by easing the pressure on your ankles and elbows.

WITH A WALL

1. Stand with your left side facing a wall. Bend your left elbow to form a 90-degree angle with your arm and place your left forearm against the wall at shoulder level.

2. Step 1 to 2 feet away from the wall and anchor your body with your forearm and feet. Hold this position for 30 seconds. Repeat these steps with your right side facing the wall.

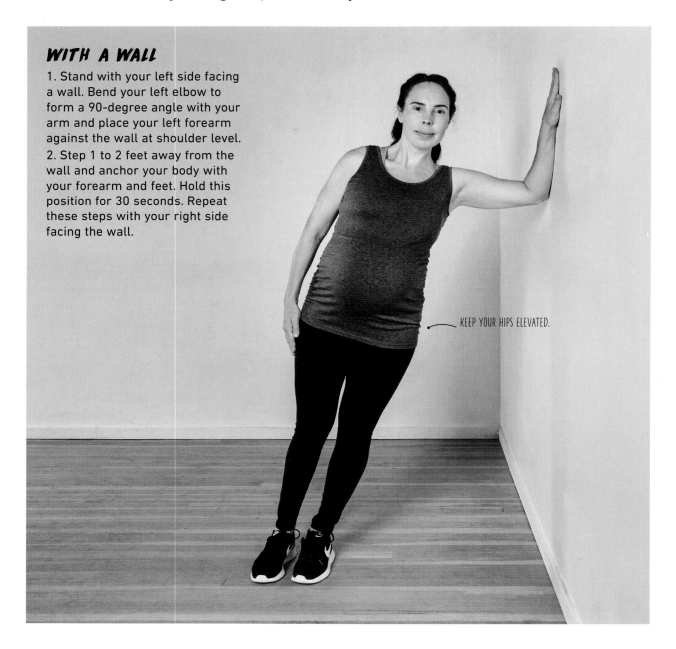

KEEP YOUR HIPS ELEVATED.

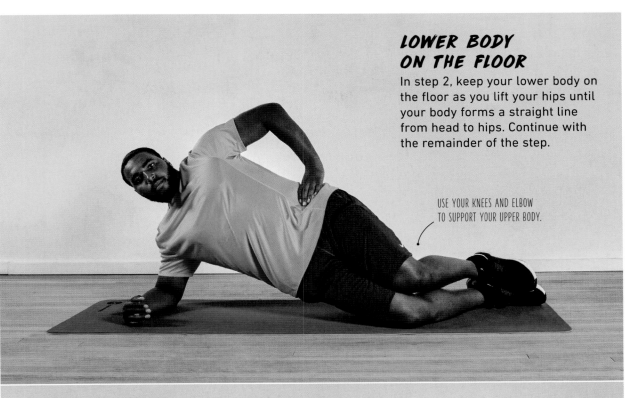

LOWER BODY ON THE FLOOR

In step 2, keep your lower body on the floor as you lift your hips until your body forms a straight line from head to hips. Continue with the remainder of the step.

USE YOUR KNEES AND ELBOW TO SUPPORT YOUR UPPER BODY.

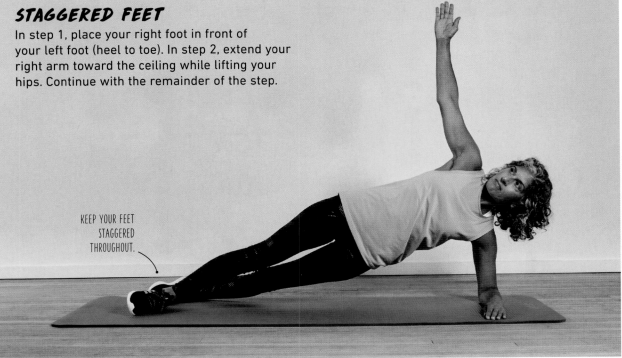

STAGGERED FEET

In step 1, place your right foot in front of your left foot (heel to toe). In step 2, extend your right arm toward the ceiling while lifting your hips. Continue with the remainder of the step.

KEEP YOUR FEET STAGGERED THROUGHOUT.

THEA HILL

I'm a mom to three young boys, a wife, a high school math teacher, an amputee, and an athlete. I've been an amputee since birth, but growing up, I wasn't particularly athletic. I learned to swim, bike, and ski, but I didn't participate in any organized team sports. It wasn't until university, where I started gaining a bit of weight, that I started to focus more on my health and exercise goals. I started by working out at the gym, but I was motivated to begin running after seeing how much my aunt, uncle, and cousins loved it. I didn't love it, but I stuck with it because it produced results and made me feel so good afterward!

At first, it was difficult because I was running on the same prosthetic leg I wore for everyday use. The ankle wasn't meant for the jarring motion of running and would keep breaking. So each time it broke, I'd have to wait until my leg was fixed until I could run again. After a while, I had a leg made purely for recreational purposes (this is the one I'm wearing in the book!), and then later, once I decided to try long-distance running, I asked for a leg that had a flex foot. With this leg, I've run countless 5K and 10K races as well as two half-marathons. At the same time I was discovering running, I also began playing para ice hockey. I had previously never considered myself to be part of the disabled community, but this sport has allowed me to meet so many differently abled people and has opened me up to friendships I'd have otherwise never had.

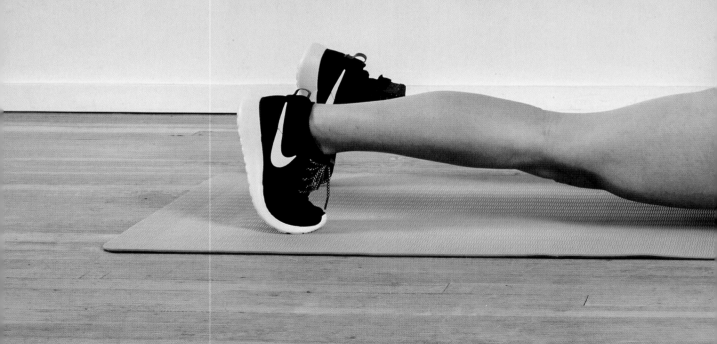

While playing para ice hockey, I realized the importance of weight training in addition to cardiovascular activities. It's necessary to have a strong core and arms, and of course, after having my children, my core was also something I wanted to strengthen. (It's a work in progress!) Exercises such as the ones in this book are perfect for someone just starting out as well as someone experienced at the gym. For example, mountain climber is an exercise I'm just not able to do in its original form, but modified with a chair or a wall— suddenly, I can actually do it! Push-ups are probably my favorite exercise. They're perfect for strengthening my arm muscles, but they're also such a great complete body exercise.

At this point in my life, exercise is one of my biggest priorities. For me, it's not about numbers on a scale or losing weight. It's about feeling strong. I love to start my day with a workout or a run. At my school, we have a group of teachers that meets before work to work out together. It's been a great way to make friends with colleagues I wouldn't have otherwise been close to and it's a place to push ourselves and try new things. Exercising helps me be a better mom because it allows me to carve out time for me and, in turn, become more patient with my children. I love being a good example for my kids and I can't wait for the day when they want to go on a run with me, although because I'm a pretty slow runner, they'll probably be miles ahead of me!

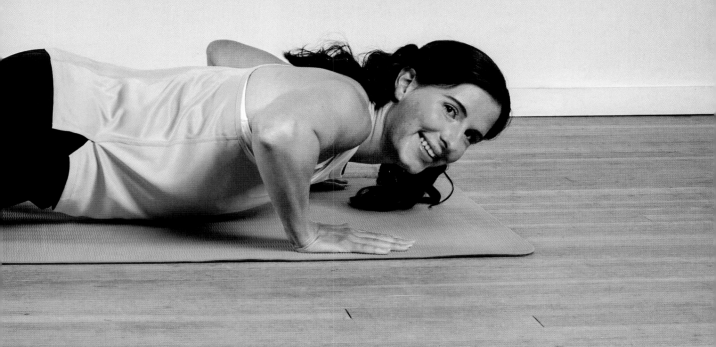

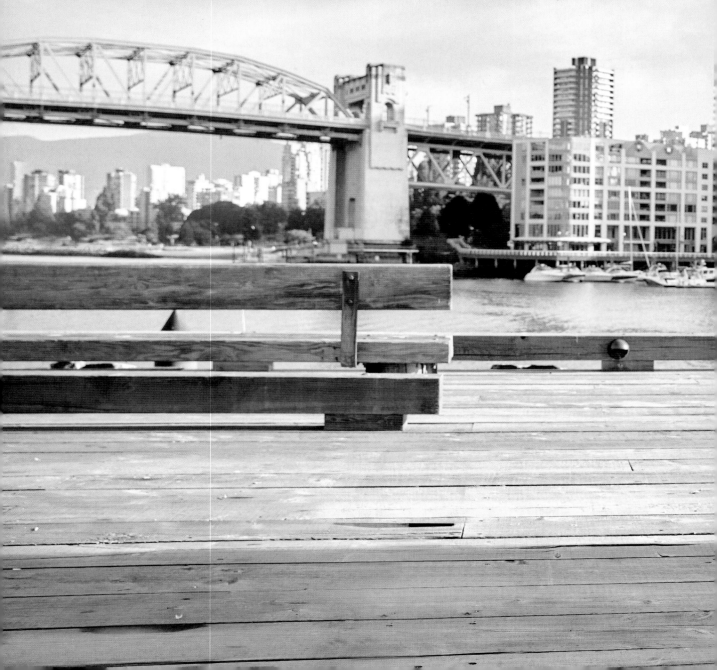

CHAPTER 3
LOWER BODY & CARDIO

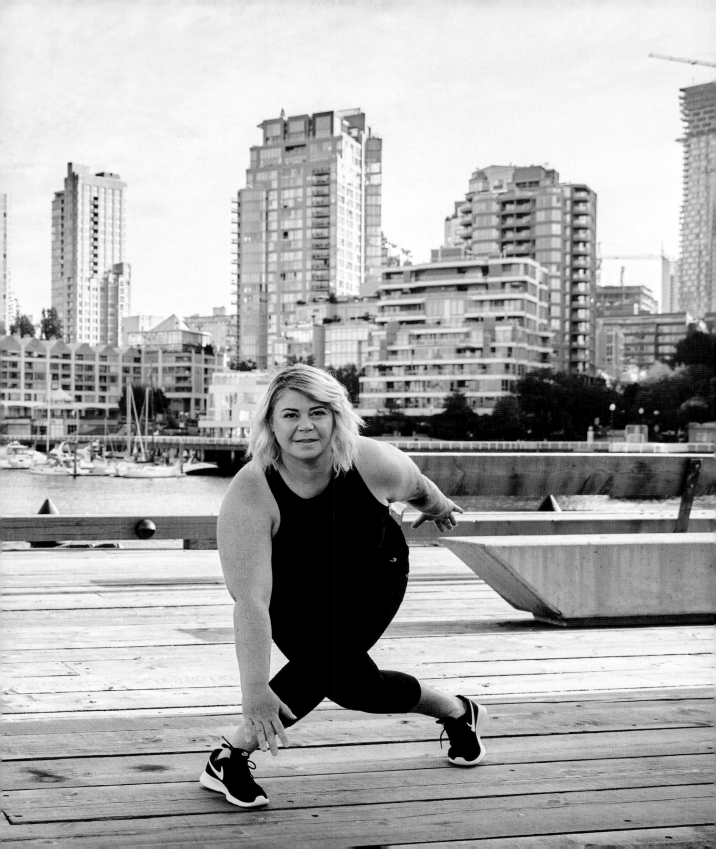

SQUAT

Squats are one of the most popular exercises and they're a mainstay in most fitness programs because of their effectiveness. They're a great way to work the front and back of your legs by targeting the quadriceps and glutes.

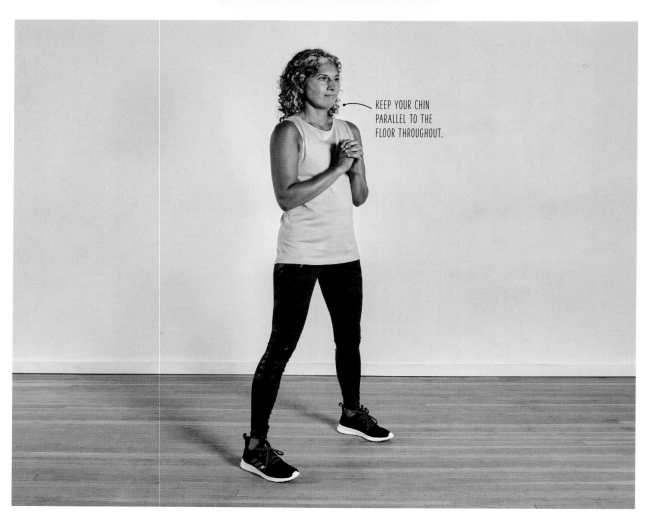

KEEP YOUR CHIN PARALLEL TO THE FLOOR THROUGHOUT.

1 Stand with your feet a little wider than shoulder width. Clasp your hands in front of your chest.

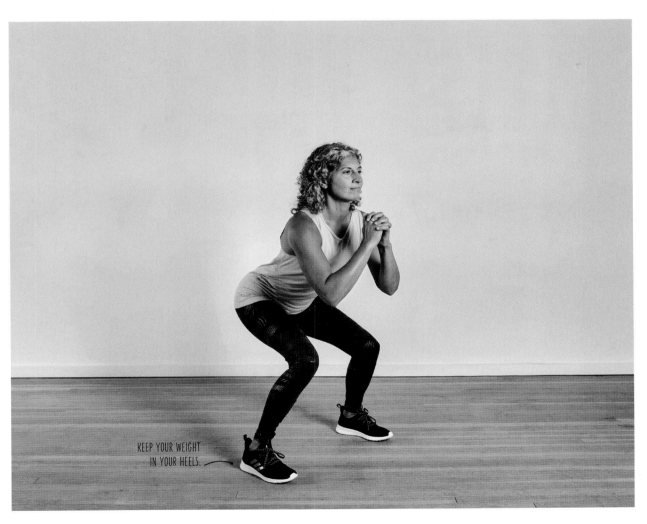

KEEP YOUR WEIGHT
IN YOUR HEELS.

2 Bend your knees to slowly lower your hips backward to form a 90-degree angle with your legs. Pause, then return to standing. Repeat this step 8 to 10 times.

// SQUAT //
VARIATIONS

Use a chair, ball, or wall to help you slowly train the body to require no assistance as you work up to the classic squat.

WITH A CHAIR

1. Stand facing away from the seat of a chair. Place your feet a little wider than shoulder width. Clasp your hands in front of your chest.

2. Slowly lower your hips toward the seat of the chair until the back of your legs just touch the chair. Pause, then return to standing. Repeat this step 8 to 10 times.

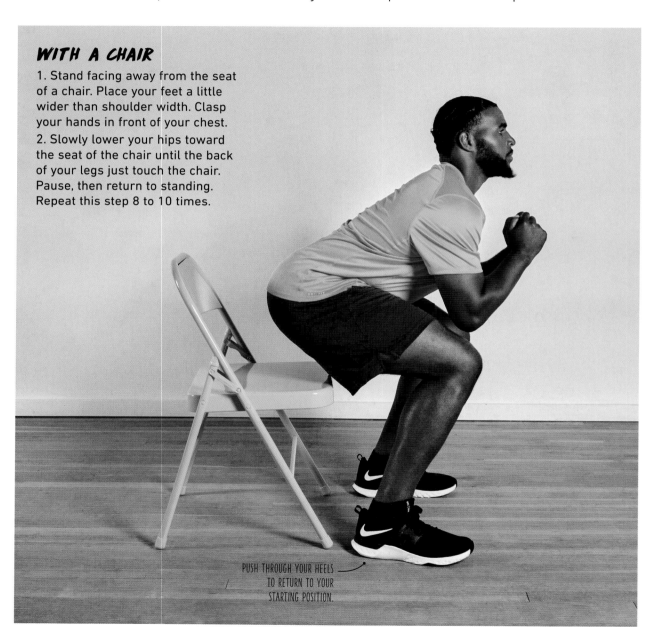

PUSH THROUGH YOUR HEELS TO RETURN TO YOUR STARTING POSITION.

WITH A WALL

1. Stand facing about 1 foot away from a wall and clasp your hands in front of your chest.

2. Slowly lower your hips backward until they touch the wall. Hold this position for 2 to 3 seconds, then return to standing. Repeat this step 8 to 10 times.

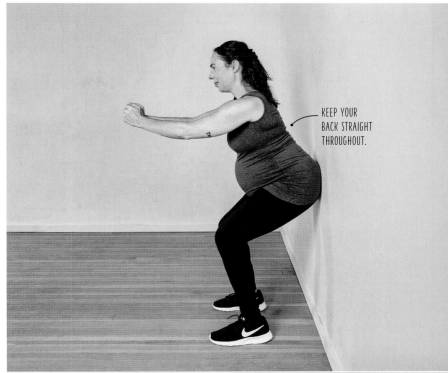

KEEP YOUR BACK STRAIGHT THROUGHOUT.

WITH A STABILITY BALL

1. Stand facing away from a wall with your feet a little wider than shoulder width. Place a stability ball against the wall and at your lower back. Clasp your hands in front of your chest.

2. Bend your knees to form a 45-degree angle with your legs. Allow the stability ball to slowly roll from your lower back to your upper back. Pause, then return to standing. Repeat this step 8 to 10 times.

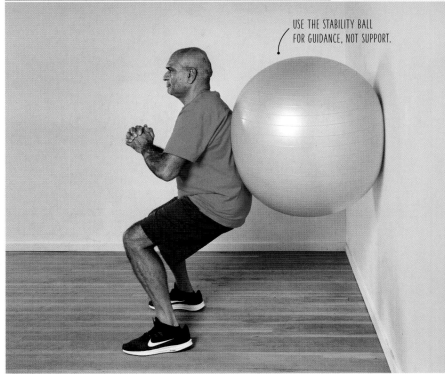

USE THE STABILITY BALL FOR GUIDANCE, NOT SUPPORT.

HIP THRUST

Your glutes develop power in the backside of your body for walking and running. Hip thrusts can help develop the glute muscles in your buttocks. This exercise is a great alternative to a squat if you have problematic knees.

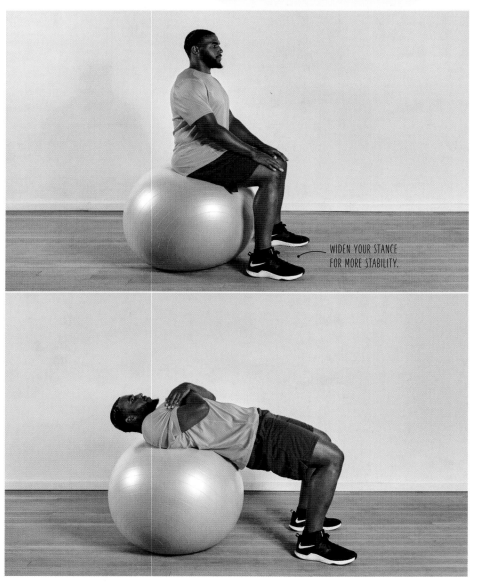

WIDEN YOUR STANCE FOR MORE STABILITY.

1 Sit on a stability ball and place your feet flat on the floor. Rest your hands on your legs.

2 Walk your feet forward until the stability ball reaches your upper back and shoulders. Lift your hips until they align with your torso.

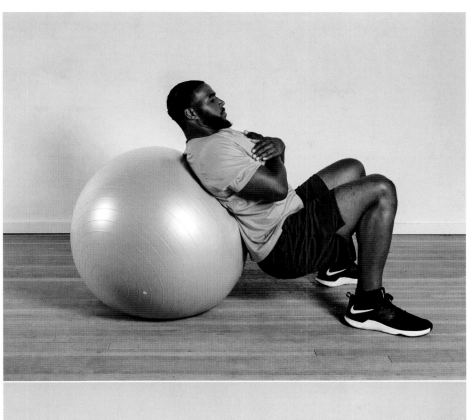

3 Lower your hips to form a 45-degree angle with your legs.

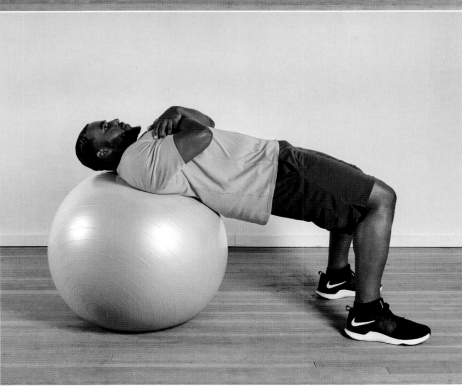

4 Drive your hips up until your legs align with your torso. Pause, then repeat these last two steps 8 to 10 times.

// HIP THRUST //

VARIATIONS

Perform this exercise against a wall or add variety
by performing the thrusts on the floor.

WITH A WALL

1. Stand with your upper back flat against a wall.
Walk your feet forward 2 steps. (Change the
intensity of this exercise by standing closer or
farther away from the wall.) Relax your arms at
your sides.

2. Slowly lower your hips backward until your
buttocks touch the wall.

3. Push your hips away from the wall. Pause,
then return your hips to the wall. Repeat this
step 8 to 10 times.

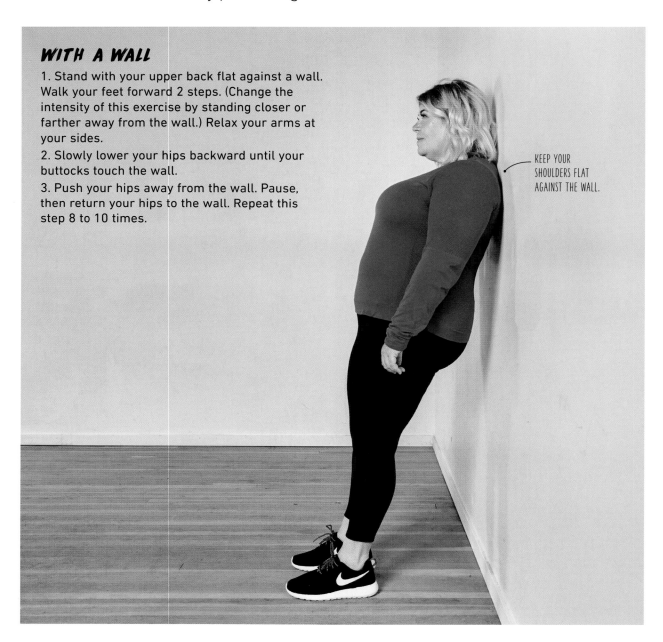

KEEP YOUR
SHOULDERS FLAT
AGAINST THE WALL.

ON THE FLOOR—BOTH LEGS

1. Lie on your back on the floor and bend your knees to place your feet flat on the floor. Relax your arms at your sides.

2. Push through your hands and feet to raise your hips off the floor. Pause, then return your hips to the floor. Repeat this step 8 to 10 times.

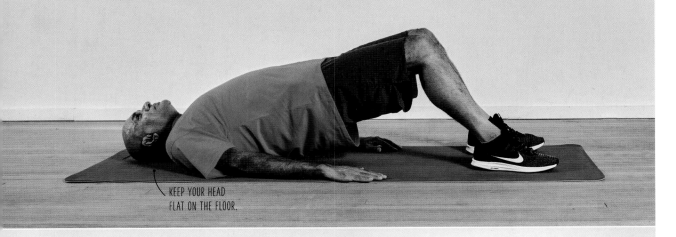

KEEP YOUR HEAD
FLAT ON THE FLOOR.

ON THE FLOOR—SINGLE LEG

1. Lie on your back on the floor and bend your knees to form a 45-degree angle with your legs. Relax your arms at your sides.

2. Lift your hips off the floor and extend your left leg toward the ceiling until aligned with your right thigh.

3. Lower your hips to the floor and keep your left leg extended. Pause, then lift your hips. Repeat this step 8 to 10 times. Repeat these steps with your right leg extended.

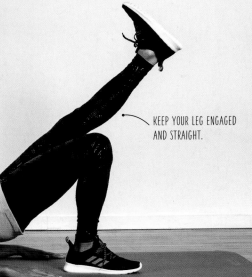

KEEP YOUR LEG ENGAGED
AND STRAIGHT.

PUSH THROUGH YOUR FOOT
TO ELEVATE YOUR HIPS.

REVERSE LUNGE

If you're looking for an introduction to lunges, a reverse lunge tends to be a little more forgiving to your knees and balance than the standard lunge. Stepping backward in this exercise stabilizes the body with less tension than the forward lunge.

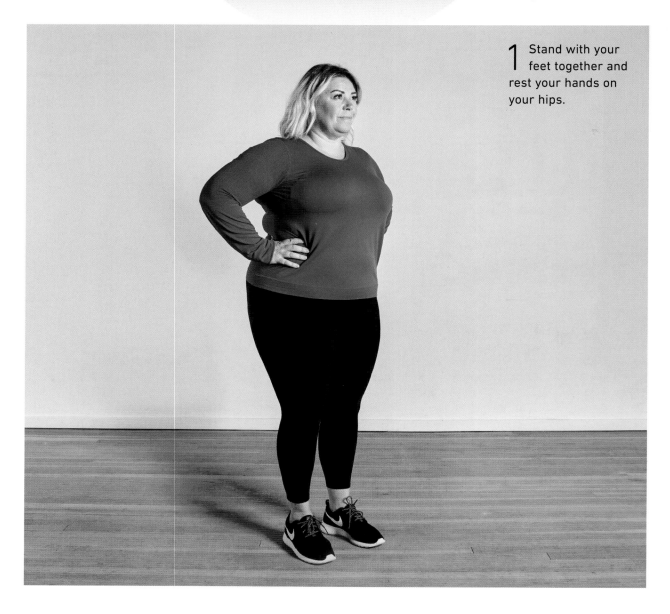

1 Stand with your feet together and rest your hands on your hips.

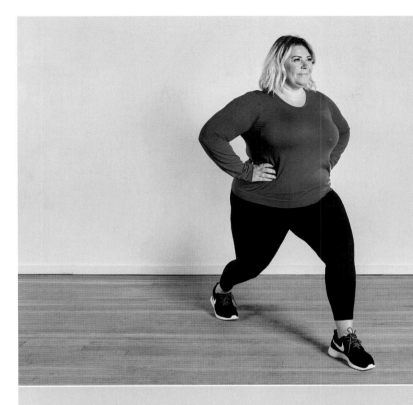

2 Step your right foot backward about 2 feet. Place the ball of your foot flat on the floor and keep your heel elevated.

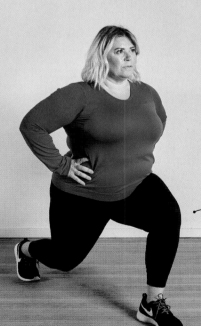

3 Bend your right knee to slowly lower your body to form a 90-degree angle with your legs. Pause, then return to standing. Repeat these last two steps 8 to 10 times. Repeat these steps with your left leg stepped backward.

ALIGN YOUR KNEE
AND ANKLE JOINTS.

// REVERSE LUNGE //

VARIATIONS

These modifications offer a shallow version, a chair option
to build balance, and a weighted variation for more challenge.

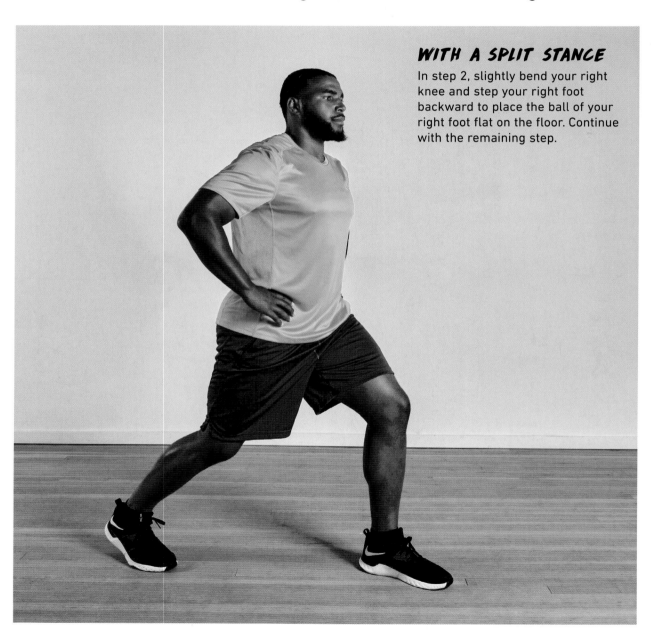

WITH A SPLIT STANCE

In step 2, slightly bend your right
knee and step your right foot
backward to place the ball of your
right foot flat on the floor. Continue
with the remaining step.

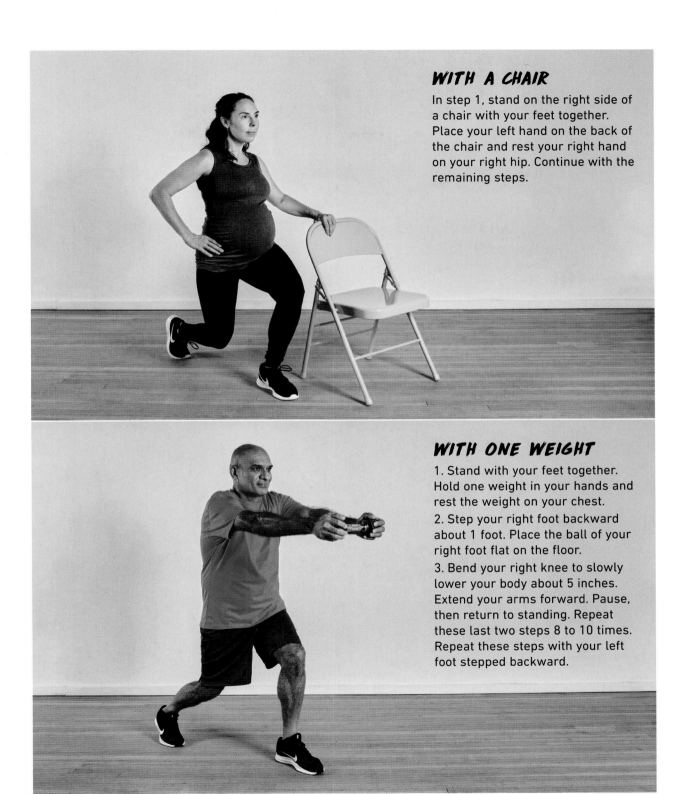

WITH A CHAIR

In step 1, stand on the right side of a chair with your feet together. Place your left hand on the back of the chair and rest your right hand on your right hip. Continue with the remaining steps.

WITH ONE WEIGHT

1. Stand with your feet together. Hold one weight in your hands and rest the weight on your chest.

2. Step your right foot backward about 1 foot. Place the ball of your right foot flat on the floor.

3. Bend your right knee to slowly lower your body about 5 inches. Extend your arms forward. Pause, then return to standing. Repeat these last two steps 8 to 10 times. Repeat these steps with your left foot stepped backward.

WALL SIT

This isometric exercise—meaning no body movement—requires some mental fortitude. Sitting against a wall can build muscular endurance, not specifically muscular strength, challenging your glutes, hamstrings, and quads while you maintain your position.

1 Stand facing 1 foot away from a wall and place your back flat against the wall. Hold one weight in your hands and rest the weight in front of your pelvis.

ENGAGE YOUR CORE THROUGHOUT FOR STABILITY.

2 Bend your knees to slowly lower your body to form a 90-degree angle with your legs.

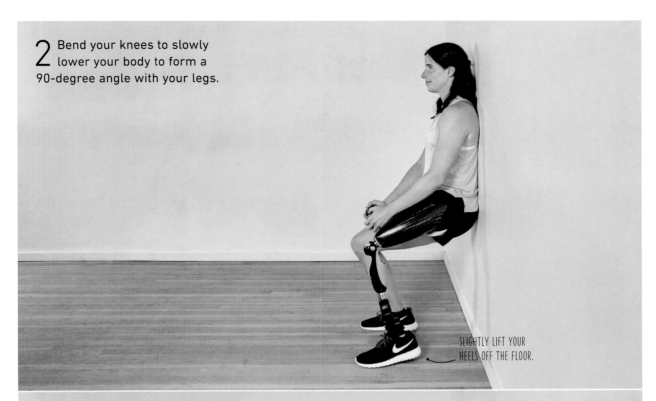

SLIGHTLY LIFT YOUR HEELS OFF THE FLOOR.

3 Extend your arms forward until parallel with the floor. Hold this position for 30 seconds.

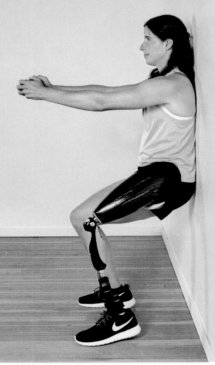

// WALL SIT //
VARIATIONS

Try the shallow version or use a chair or a stability ball
to take some pressure off your knees.

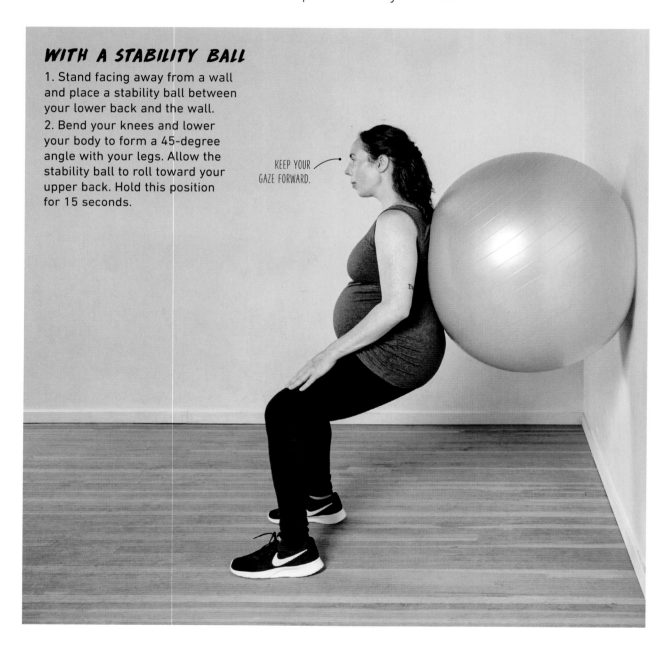

WITH A STABILITY BALL

1. Stand facing away from a wall and place a stability ball between your lower back and the wall.

2. Bend your knees and lower your body to form a 45-degree angle with your legs. Allow the stability ball to roll toward your upper back. Hold this position for 15 seconds.

KEEP YOUR GAZE FORWARD.

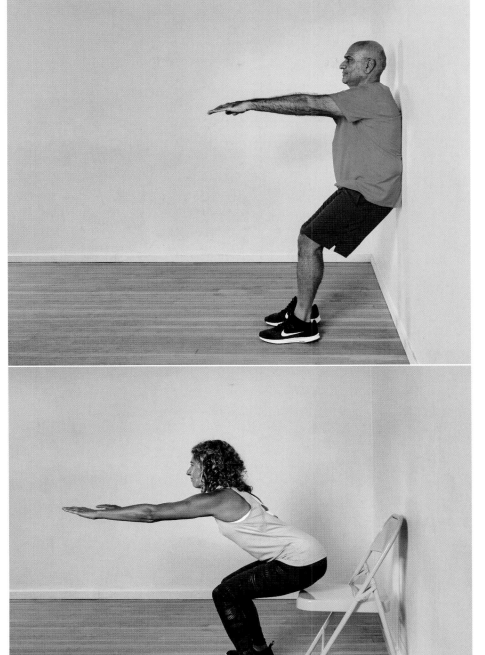

KEEP YOUR WEIGHT
IN YOUR HEELS.

SHALLOW SIT

1. Stand facing 1 foot away from a wall and place your back flat against the wall. Relax your arms at your sides.

2. Slightly bend your knees to slowly lower your body to form a 45-degree angle with your legs.

3. Extend your arms forward until parallel with the floor. Hold this position for 30 seconds.

WITH A CHAIR

1. Stand facing away from the seat of a chair and relax your arms at your sides.

2. Bend your knees to slowly lower your body until your buttocks slightly touch the seat of the chair.

3. Extend your arms forward until parallel with the floor. Hold this position for 30 seconds. (Hover 1 to 2 inches off the seat. You can sit if needed, but return to the hovering position until the time ends.)

DONKEY KICK

These movements isolate your hamstrings and they're easier on your body than other hamstring exercises. This is an excellent alternative to strengthen the back of your legs and your glutes, helping you maintain sound posture and prevent back injuries.

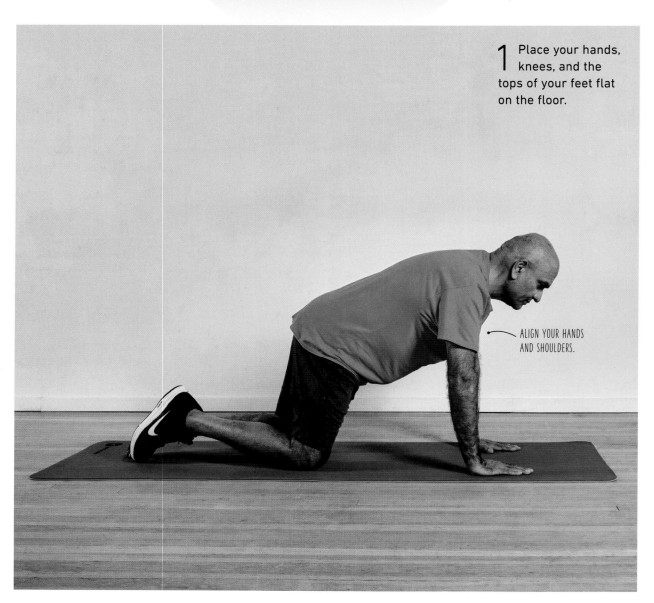

1 Place your hands, knees, and the tops of your feet flat on the floor.

ALIGN YOUR HANDS AND SHOULDERS.

2 Lift your right knee and right foot off the floor to slowly extend your right leg toward the ceiling. Pause, then lower your right knee to the floor. Repeat this step 8 to 10 times. Repeat these steps with your left leg extended.

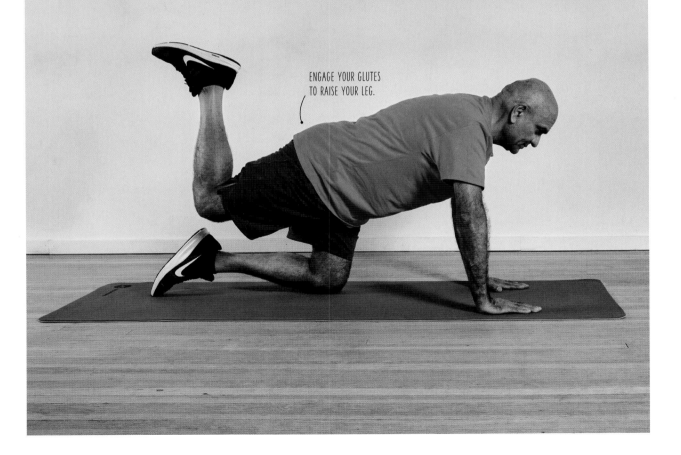

ENGAGE YOUR GLUTES TO RAISE YOUR LEG.

// DONKEY KICK //
VARIATIONS

Donkeys do kick from all angles! But you can perform this exercise by using a chair or a wall or rotating your hip for variety.

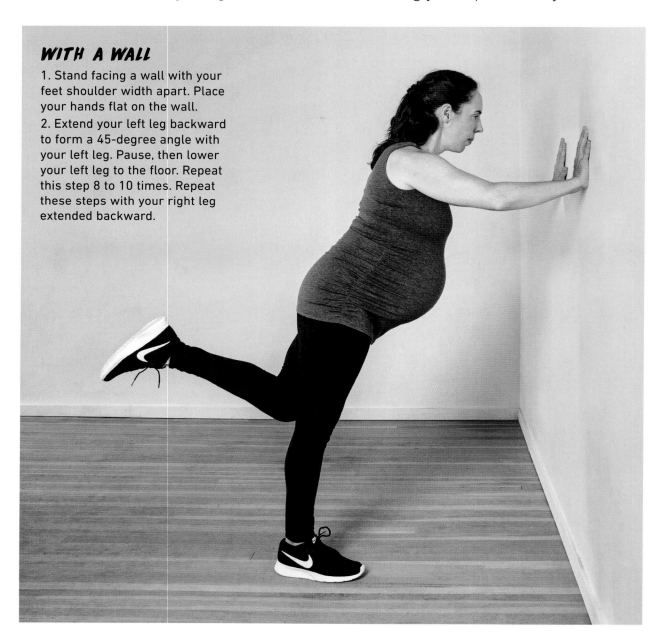

WITH A WALL

1. Stand facing a wall with your feet shoulder width apart. Place your hands flat on the wall.

2. Extend your left leg backward to form a 45-degree angle with your left leg. Pause, then lower your left leg to the floor. Repeat this step 8 to 10 times. Repeat these steps with your right leg extended backward.

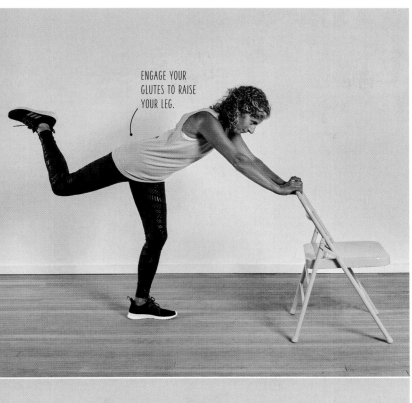

ENGAGE YOUR GLUTES TO RAISE YOUR LEG.

WITH A CHAIR

1. Stand 2 feet behind the back of a chair with your feet shoulder width apart. Place your hands on the back of the chair.

2. Bend at your waist to form a 45-degree angle with your body and extend your right leg backward. Pause, then lower your right leg until your knees align. (Keeping your leg off the floor will help you maintain your momentum.) Repeat this step 8 to 10 times. Repeat these steps with your left leg extended backward.

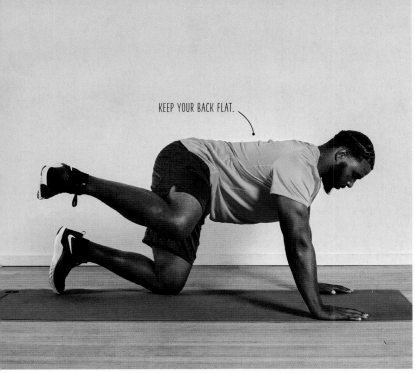

KEEP YOUR BACK FLAT.

WITH LATERAL MOVEMENTS

In step 2, extend your right leg toward your right side. Pause, then lower your right leg to the floor. Repeat this step 8 to 10 times. Repeat these steps with your left leg extended to your left side.

FAST FEET

You can add this cardio move to any exercise routine for a bit of punch to your heart rate. Although this is primarily for cardio, you'll work your calves, quadriceps, and hamstrings. Depending on the tempo of your feet, this can be advanced or beginner.

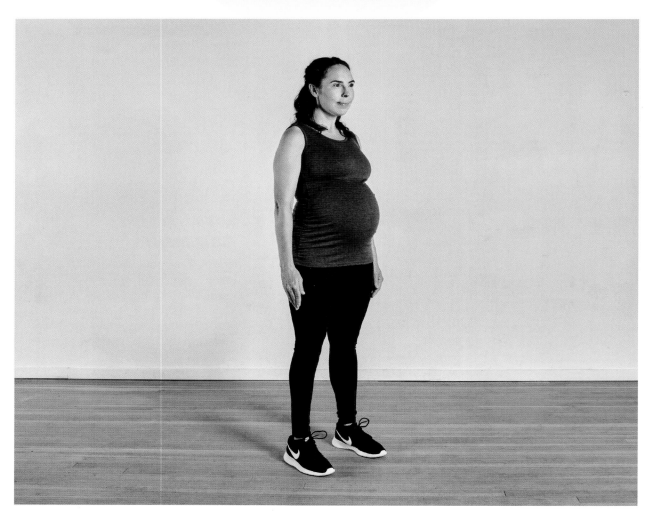

1 Stand with your feet shoulder width apart and relax your arms at your sides.

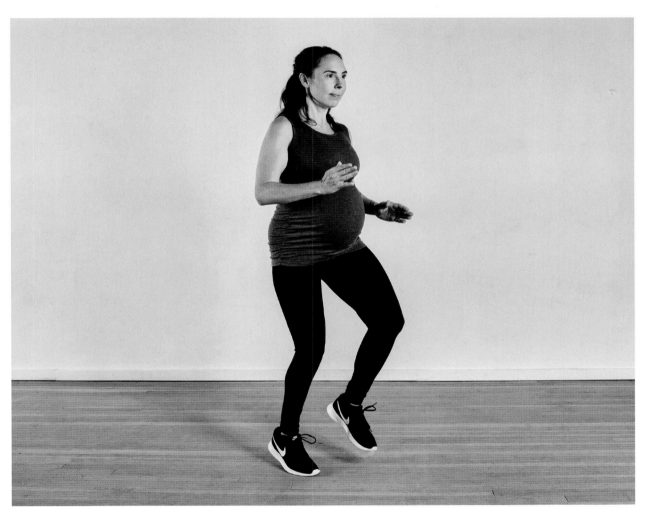

2 Push down through the balls of your feet and quickly run in place. Move your arms up and down in tandem with the momentum of your legs. Perform this step for 30 seconds.

// FAST FEET //
VARIATIONS

With these modifications, you can slow down the tempo
or change your stance or you can do this exercise while seated.

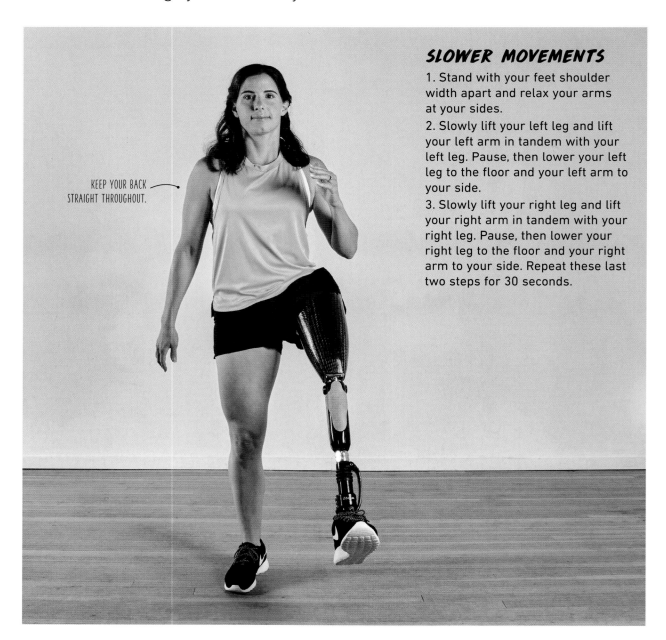

KEEP YOUR BACK
STRAIGHT THROUGHOUT.

SLOWER MOVEMENTS

1. Stand with your feet shoulder width apart and relax your arms at your sides.

2. Slowly lift your left leg and lift your left arm in tandem with your left leg. Pause, then lower your left leg to the floor and your left arm to your side.

3. Slowly lift your right leg and lift your right arm in tandem with your right leg. Pause, then lower your right leg to the floor and your right arm to your side. Repeat these last two steps for 30 seconds.

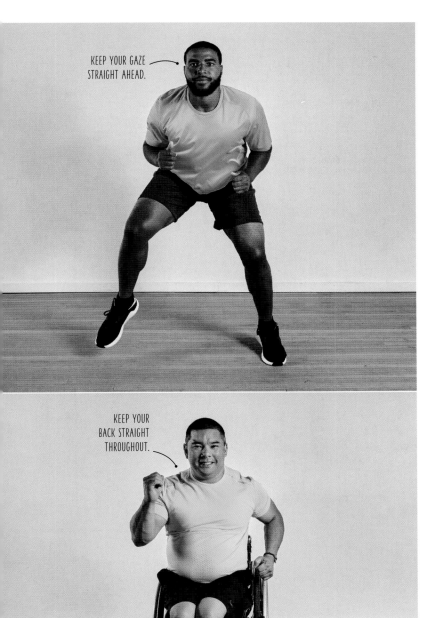

KEEP YOUR GAZE STRAIGHT AHEAD.

CHANGING YOUR STANCE

In step 2, with every 5 foot movements, alternate between widening and narrowing your running stance.

KEEP YOUR BACK STRAIGHT THROUGHOUT.

SEATED

1. Sit in a chair and place your feet flat on the floor. Relax your arms at your sides.

2. Bend your right elbow and lift your right hand to align with your shoulders. (You can also lift your right knee toward your chest.) Pause, then lower your right arm to your side.

3. Bend your left elbow and lift your left hand to align with your shoulders. (You can also lift your left knee toward your chest.) Pause, then lower your left arm to your side. Repeat these last two steps for 30 seconds.

DEADLIFT

If you're looking to build more strength into your backside for better posture and lifting power, this is a great way to start. This exercise strengthens your hamstrings, glutes, and lower and upper back muscles, relying heavily on core strength.

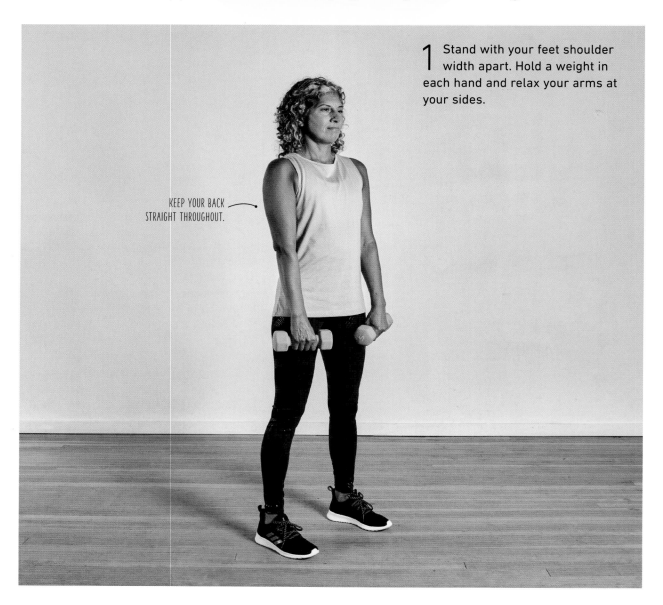

1 Stand with your feet shoulder width apart. Hold a weight in each hand and relax your arms at your sides.

KEEP YOUR BACK STRAIGHT THROUGHOUT.

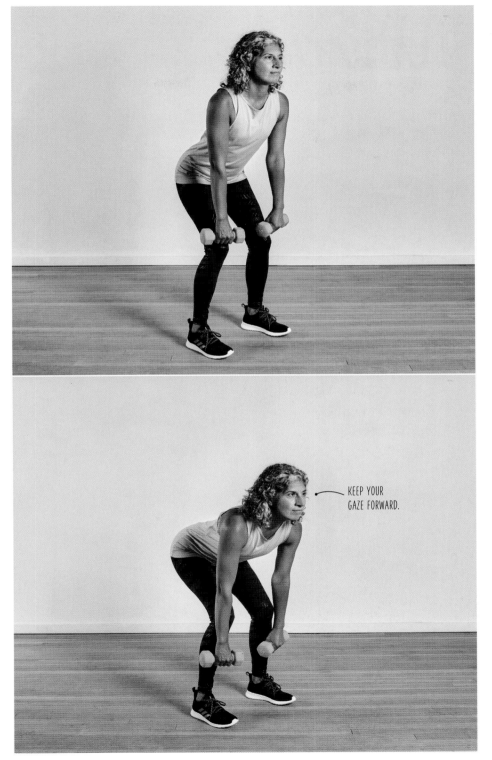

KEEP YOUR
GAZE FORWARD.

2 Slowly bend at your waist and lower the weights to your knees.

3 Bend your knees to lower your body into a squat. Lower your arms until the weights reach your shins. Pause, then return to standing. Repeat these last two steps 8 to 10 times.

// DEADLIFT //
VARIATIONS

This exercise can take some practice. These options offer ways to stay in form with a wall, staggered legs, or no weights.

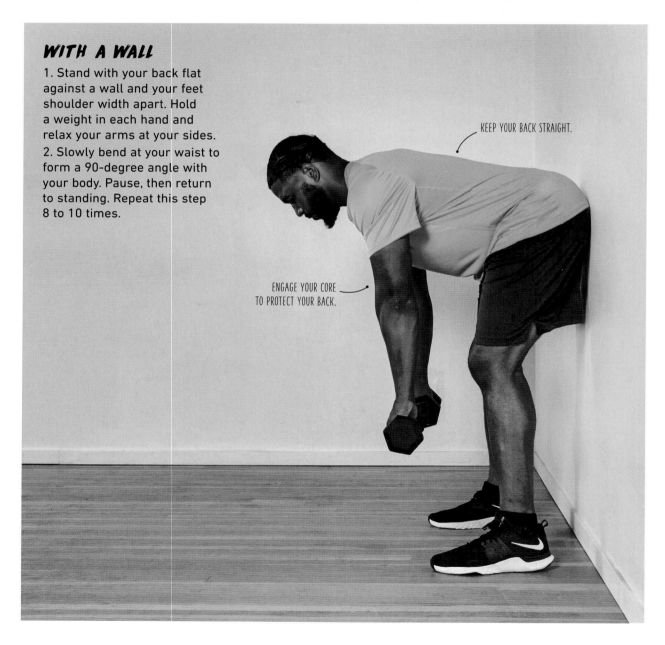

WITH A WALL

1. Stand with your back flat against a wall and your feet shoulder width apart. Hold a weight in each hand and relax your arms at your sides.

2. Slowly bend at your waist to form a 90-degree angle with your body. Pause, then return to standing. Repeat this step 8 to 10 times.

KEEP YOUR BACK STRAIGHT.

ENGAGE YOUR CORE TO PROTECT YOUR BACK.

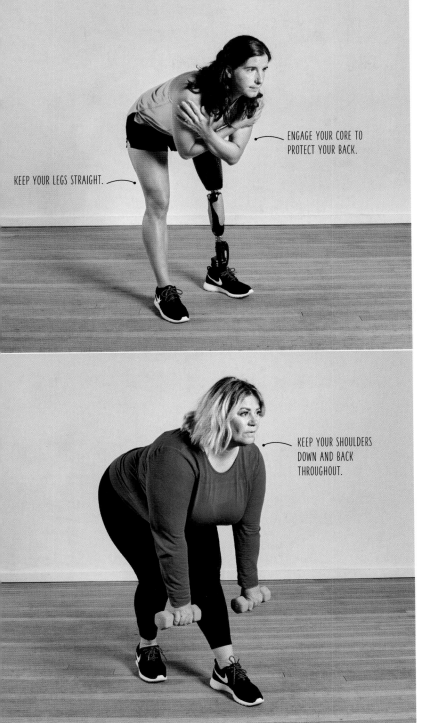

ENGAGE YOUR CORE TO PROTECT YOUR BACK.

KEEP YOUR LEGS STRAIGHT.

KEEP YOUR SHOULDERS DOWN AND BACK THROUGHOUT.

WITHOUT WEIGHTS

1. Stand with your feet shoulder width apart and cross your arms in front of your chest.

2. Slowly bend at your waist to form a 90-degree angle with your body. Pause, then return to standing. Repeat this step 8 to 10 times.

WITH A SPLIT STANCE

1. Stand with your feet shoulder width apart. Hold a weight in each hand and relax your arms at your sides.

2. Step your left foot forward about 1 foot and place your left foot flat on the floor.

3. Slowly bend at your waist and slowly bend your right knee to form a 45-degree angle with your right leg. Lower the weights toward your shins. Pause, then slowly return to standing. Repeat these last two steps 8 to 10 times. Repeat these steps with your right foot stepped forward and your left knee bent.

LATERAL LEG RAISE

This exercise targets the abductor and glute medius muscles, which stabilize your legs when walking or standing. Adding a squat at a quick tempo allows you to also enjoy the benefits of cardio. (For less cardio, slow down the tempo.)

1 Stand with your feet shoulder width apart and clasp your hands in front of your chest.

2 Bend your knees to form a 45-degree angle with your legs and push your hips backward to lower into a squat.

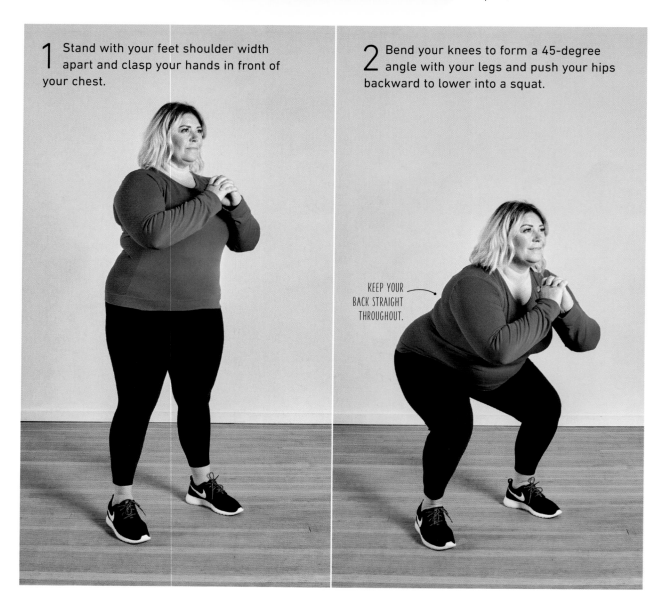

KEEP YOUR BACK STRAIGHT THROUGHOUT.

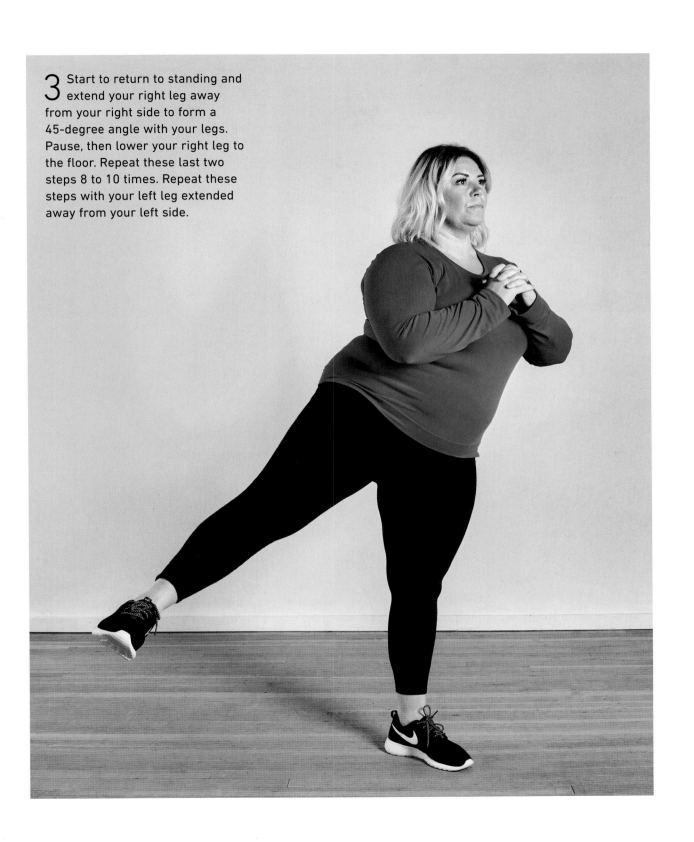

3 Start to return to standing and extend your right leg away from your right side to form a 45-degree angle with your legs. Pause, then lower your right leg to the floor. Repeat these last two steps 8 to 10 times. Repeat these steps with your left leg extended away from your left side.

// LATERAL LEG RAISE //
VARIATIONS

While there are many ways to raise your leg, these modifications offer ways to perform the exercise if you have any knee issues.

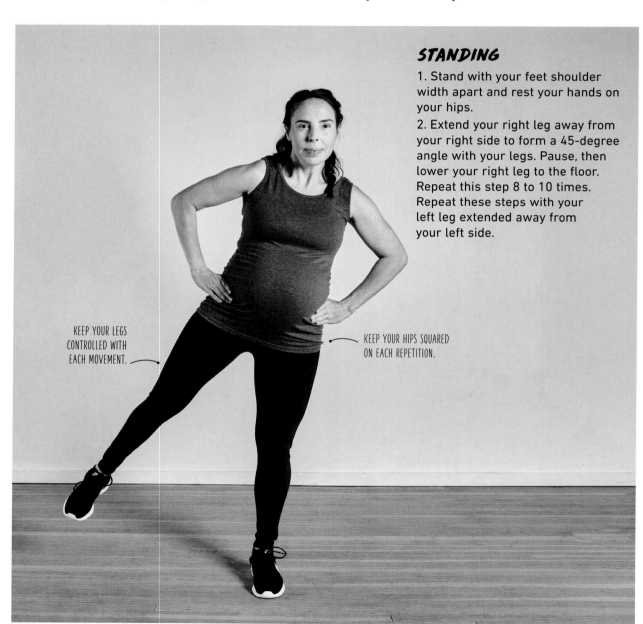

STANDING

1. Stand with your feet shoulder width apart and rest your hands on your hips.
2. Extend your right leg away from your right side to form a 45-degree angle with your legs. Pause, then lower your right leg to the floor. Repeat this step 8 to 10 times. Repeat these steps with your left leg extended away from your left side.

KEEP YOUR LEGS CONTROLLED WITH EACH MOVEMENT.

KEEP YOUR HIPS SQUARED ON EACH REPETITION.

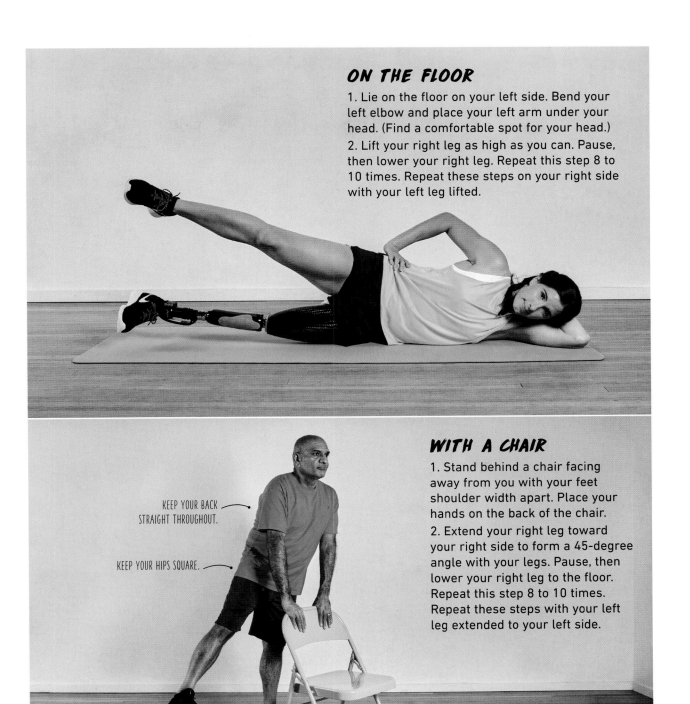

ON THE FLOOR

1. Lie on the floor on your left side. Bend your left elbow and place your left arm under your head. (Find a comfortable spot for your head.)

2. Lift your right leg as high as you can. Pause, then lower your right leg. Repeat this step 8 to 10 times. Repeat these steps on your right side with your left leg lifted.

WITH A CHAIR

1. Stand behind a chair facing away from you with your feet shoulder width apart. Place your hands on the back of the chair.

2. Extend your right leg toward your right side to form a 45-degree angle with your legs. Pause, then lower your right leg to the floor. Repeat this step 8 to 10 times. Repeat these steps with your left leg extended to your left side.

KEEP YOUR BACK STRAIGHT THROUGHOUT.

KEEP YOUR HIPS SQUARE.

KEEP YOUR FOOT FLAT ON THE FLOOR.

JAB & CROSS

Boxing moves are quick cardio blasts that can raise your heart rate and add speed to create high-intensity interval training workouts or to just build your cardiovascular system. Go faster for more intensity or go slowly to moderate your heart rate.

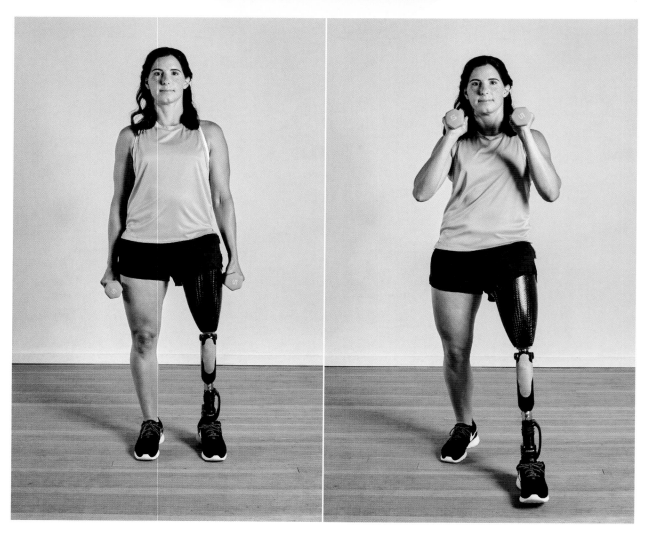

1 Stand with your feet shoulder width apart. Hold a weight in each hand and relax your arms at your sides.

2 Step your left foot forward and bend your elbows to lift the weights toward your chin.

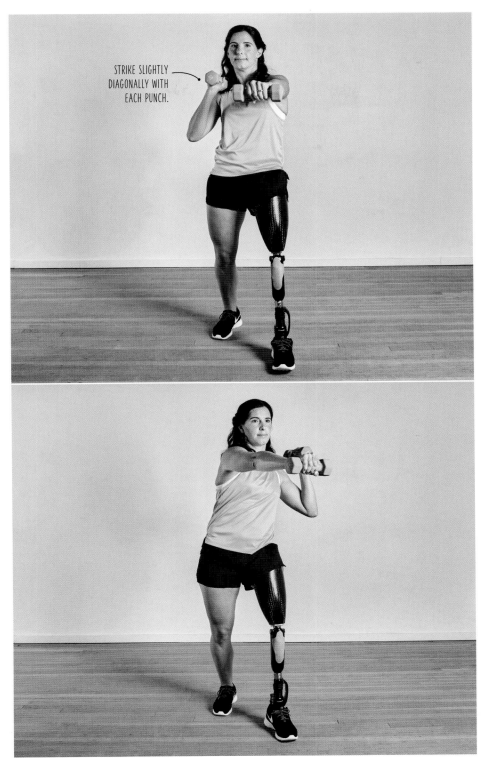

STRIKE SLIGHTLY DIAGONALLY WITH EACH PUNCH.

3 Quickly extend your left arm forward in a striking motion. Return your left hand to your chin and take two steps to your right.

4 Quickly extend your right arm forward in a striking motion. Return your right hand to your chin and take two steps to your left. Repeat these last two steps for 30 seconds.

// JAB & CROSS //
VARIATIONS

With these variations, you can manage and control your intensity by either sitting, kneeling, or standing in one position.

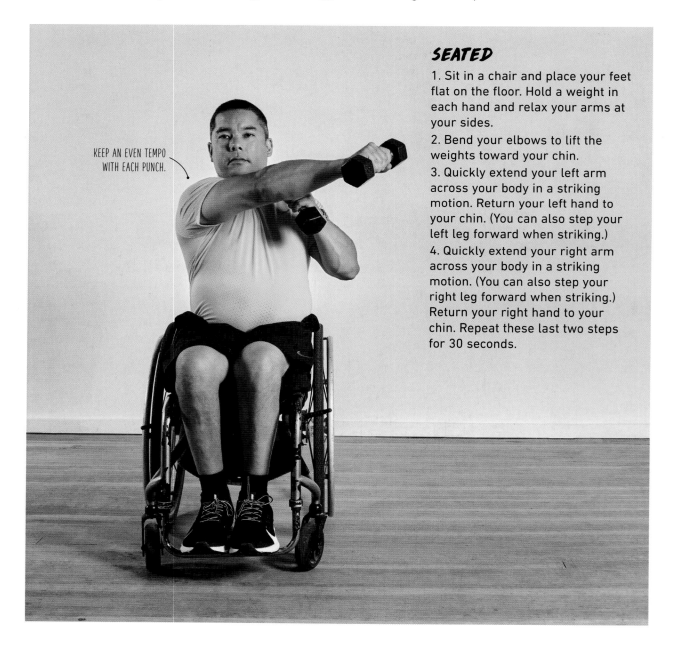

KEEP AN EVEN TEMPO WITH EACH PUNCH.

SEATED

1. Sit in a chair and place your feet flat on the floor. Hold a weight in each hand and relax your arms at your sides.

2. Bend your elbows to lift the weights toward your chin.

3. Quickly extend your left arm across your body in a striking motion. Return your left hand to your chin. (You can also step your left leg forward when striking.)

4. Quickly extend your right arm across your body in a striking motion. (You can also step your right leg forward when striking.) Return your right hand to your chin. Repeat these last two steps for 30 seconds.

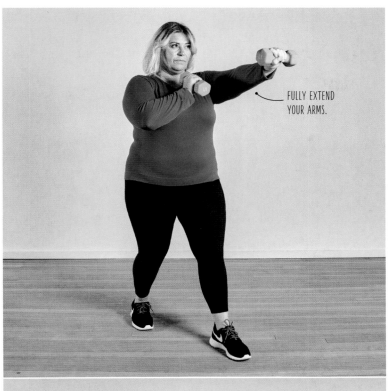

FULLY EXTEND YOUR ARMS.

STAYING STATIONARY

In steps 3 and 4, keep your feet stationary rather than taking steps with each punch.

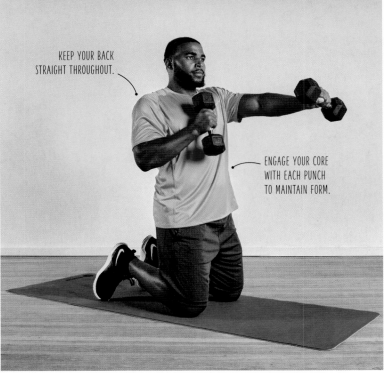

KEEP YOUR BACK STRAIGHT THROUGHOUT.

ENGAGE YOUR CORE WITH EACH PUNCH TO MAINTAIN FORM.

ON YOUR KNEES

1. Place your knees flat on the floor. Hold a weight in each hand and rest your hands in front of your chin.

2. Quickly extend your left arm forward in a striking motion. Return your left hand to your chin.

3. Quickly extend your right arm forward in a striking motion. Return your right hand to your chin. Repeat these last two steps for 30 seconds.

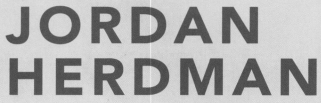

JORDAN HERDMAN

My fitness journey started at a very young age. I can remember my father taking my twin brother and me through football drills as early as 3 years old. As a kid, I didn't completely understand what I was doing—I was just having fun—but little did I know I was building a foundation that would help me later in my life.

The first time I put on shoulder pads and a helmet, I was 10. I remember getting my first tackle, hitting the ball carrier with all my strength and tackling him

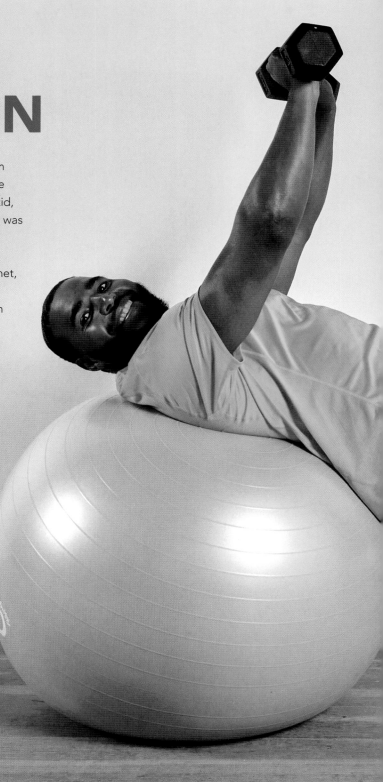

to the ground, and feeling the joy and excitement. It was at that moment I fell in love with the game and knew I was going to be a pro football player when I got older.

However, as I continued playing through high school and college, I realized how many obstacles I had to overcome to reach my dream. Less than 1% of football players make it to the professional level, and keep in mind, I was never the biggest, the strongest, or even the fastest player. The odds were definitely against me. Because of this, football taught me many life lessons: how to be resilient and that you're going to get knocked down—just like a tackle in football—but you can't give up. You must will yourself back up, knock the dust off, and get ready for the next play.

I was even told many times I could never be a pro football player because I was too small or too slow.

However, I learned that the same people who said those things didn't measure my heart and how hard I worked. So I didn't worry about the negative comments but instead believed in myself and put in the effort and stayed persistent. Now that I've been a pro football player in the Canadian Football League since 2017, I can say: "Don't ever give up or let anyone tell you that you can't achieve your dream—no matter how hard it might seem."

When I'm not playing football, I speak with at-risk youth about what I've learned, such as making good choices, setting goals, and staying active through playing sports. I'm also a personal trainer in my spare time for my business "The Kings of Hustle," which helps young football players reach their football aspirations—just like I did.

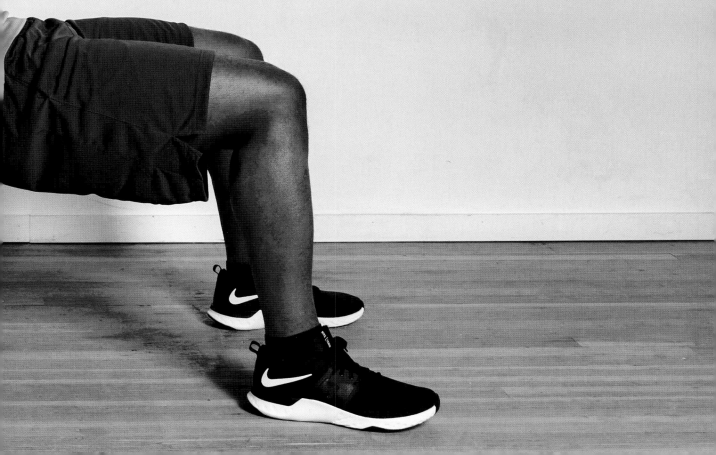

SINGLE-LEG CALF RAISE

Because your calves hold up most of your weight, they deserve some attention. This exercise helps develop the soleus and gastrocnemius muscles—critical for walking, running, and jumping because they pull the heels up for forward movement.

1 Stand with your left foot flat on the floor and bend your right knee to form a 90-degree angle with your right leg. Relax your arms at your sides.

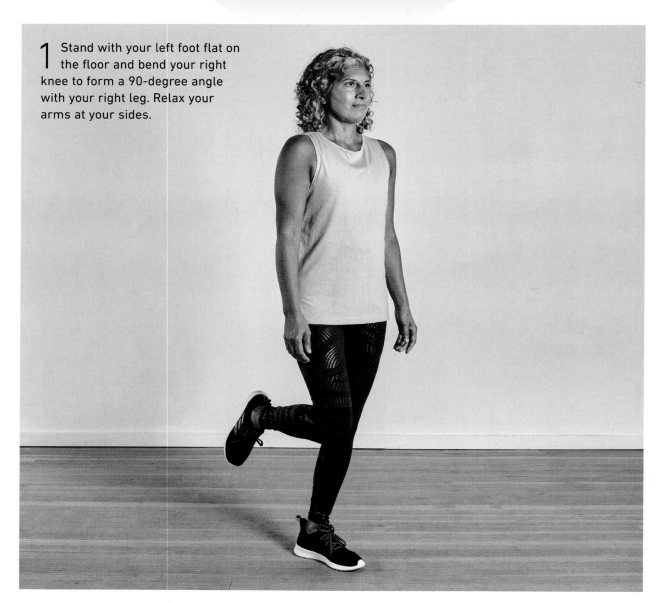

2 Lift your left heel off the floor and push up from the ball of your left foot to elevate your body. Pause, then lower your left heel to the floor. Repeat this step 8 to 10 times. Repeat these steps with your right foot flat on the floor and your left leg bent.

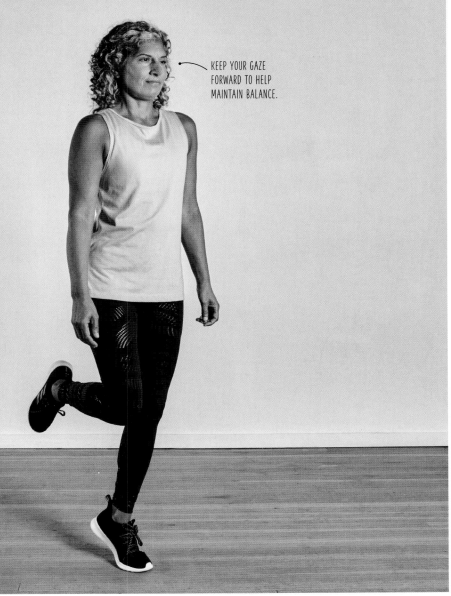

KEEP YOUR GAZE FORWARD TO HELP MAINTAIN BALANCE.

// SINGLE-LEG CALF RAISE //
VARIATIONS

One great way to modify this exercise is to make it a double calf raise because this helps with balance.

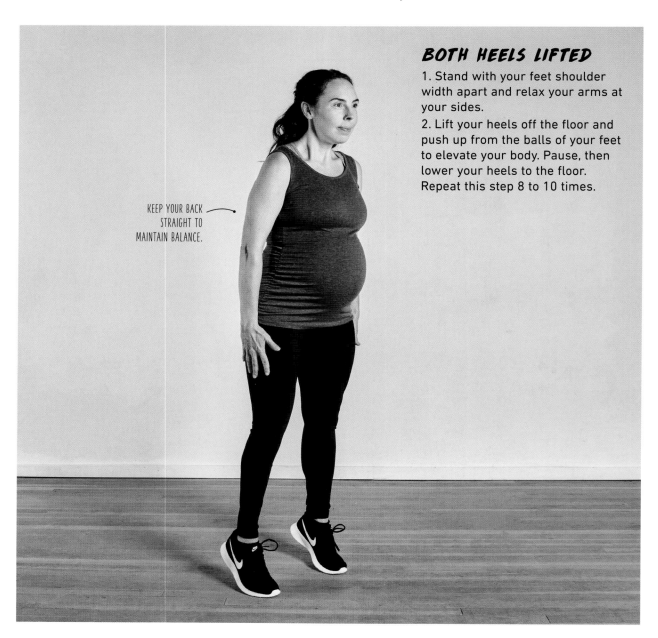

BOTH HEELS LIFTED

1. Stand with your feet shoulder width apart and relax your arms at your sides.
2. Lift your heels off the floor and push up from the balls of your feet to elevate your body. Pause, then lower your heels to the floor. Repeat this step 8 to 10 times.

KEEP YOUR BACK STRAIGHT TO MAINTAIN BALANCE.

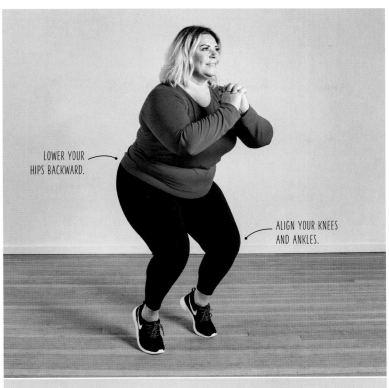

LOWER YOUR HIPS BACKWARD.

ALIGN YOUR KNEES AND ANKLES.

SQUATTING & WITH BOTH HEELS LIFTED

1. Stand with your feet shoulder width apart. Clasp your hands in front of your chest.

2. Bend your knees and lift your heels off the floor. Push up from the balls of your feet to elevate your body. Pause, then lower your heels to the floor. Repeat this step 8 to 10 times.

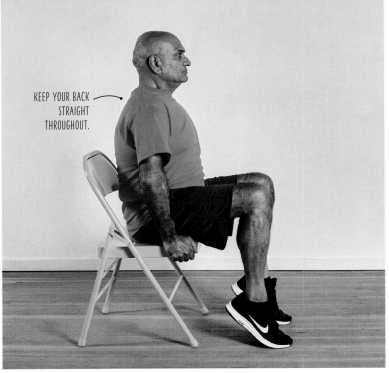

KEEP YOUR BACK STRAIGHT THROUGHOUT.

SEATED

1. Sit in a chair and place your feet flat on the floor. Place your hands on the sides of the seat of the chair.

2. Lift your heels off the floor and balance your legs on the balls of your feet. Pause, then lower your heels to the floor. Repeat this step 8 to 10 times.

SQUAT KICK

Kicking motions offer a simple way to work your leg muscles, especially your quadriceps and hip flexors. But kicks can also elevate your heart rate while offering a cardio jolt to any workout. Plus, they add fun and variety to any routine.

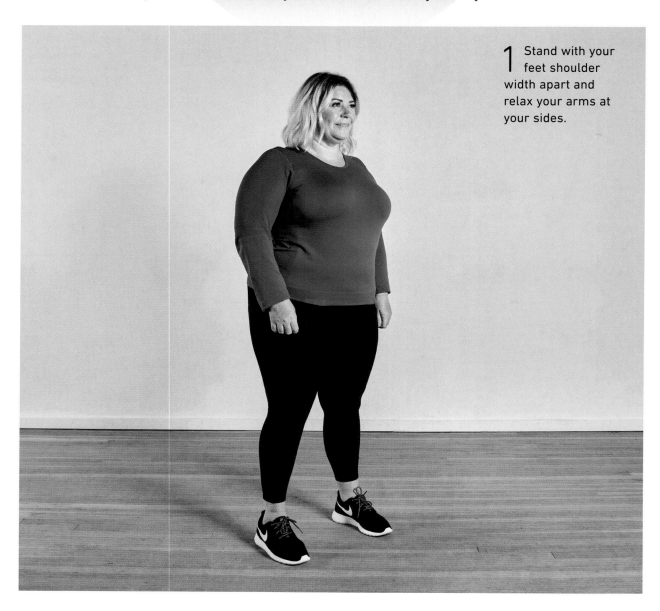

1 Stand with your feet shoulder width apart and relax your arms at your sides.

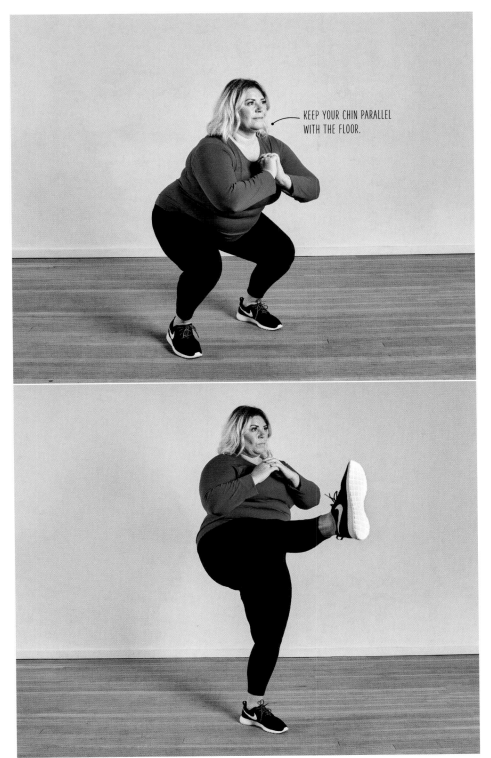

KEEP YOUR CHIN PARALLEL WITH THE FLOOR.

2 Bend your knees to slowly lower your body to form a 90-degree angle with your legs. Clasp your hands in front of your chest.

3 As you begin to stand up, kick your right leg forward until your right leg is parallel with the floor. Pause, then lower your right leg to the floor. Repeat these last two steps 8 to 10 times. Repeat these steps with your left leg.

// SQUAT KICK //
VARIATIONS

Modify this exercise to make it more accessible
by removing the squat or using a chair for assistance.

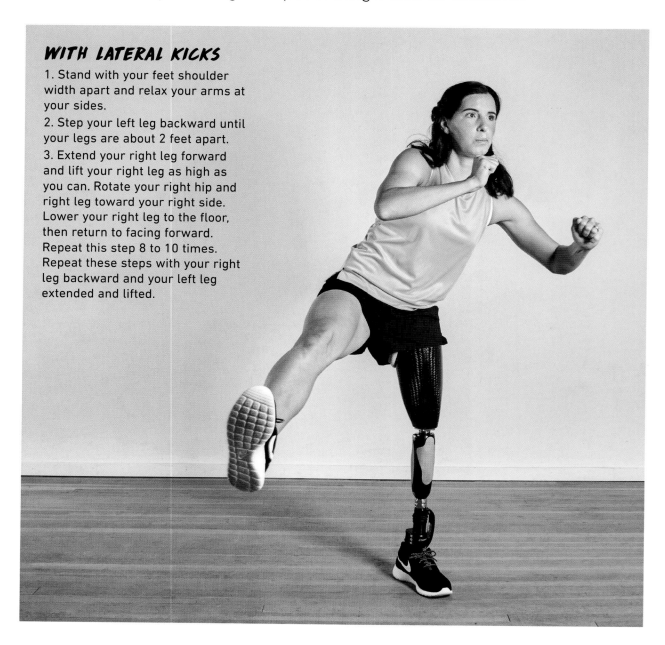

WITH LATERAL KICKS

1. Stand with your feet shoulder width apart and relax your arms at your sides.

2. Step your left leg backward until your legs are about 2 feet apart.

3. Extend your right leg forward and lift your right leg as high as you can. Rotate your right hip and right leg toward your right side. Lower your right leg to the floor, then return to facing forward. Repeat this step 8 to 10 times. Repeat these steps with your right leg backward and your left leg extended and lifted.

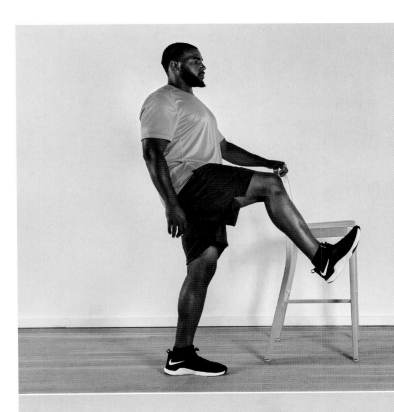

WITH A CHAIR

1. Stand on the right side of a chair. Place your left hand on the back of the chair and relax your right arm at your side.

2. Bend your right knee and lift your right leg to hip height. Kick your right foot straight out. Pause, then lower your leg to the floor. Repeat this step 8 to 10 times. Repeat these steps on the left side of the chair with your left knee and left foot.

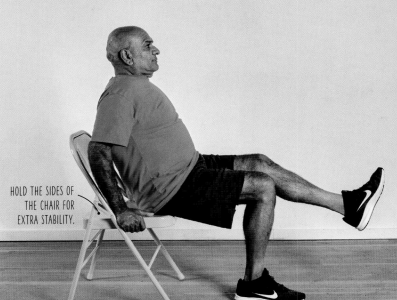

HOLD THE SIDES OF THE CHAIR FOR EXTRA STABILITY.

SEATED

1. Sit on the edge of the seat of a chair and place your feet flat on the floor. Relax your arms at your sides.

2. Lift your left leg until aligned with your left hip. Kick your left foot straight out. Pause, then lower your left leg to the floor. Repeat this step 8 to 10 times. Repeat these steps with your right leg.

SPEED SKATING

Incorporating this exercise into your fitness routine adds cardio, stamina, and endurance. Skating movements also build strength in your quadriceps, glutes, hamstrings, and calves. Plus, they offer a good sweat while working through them.

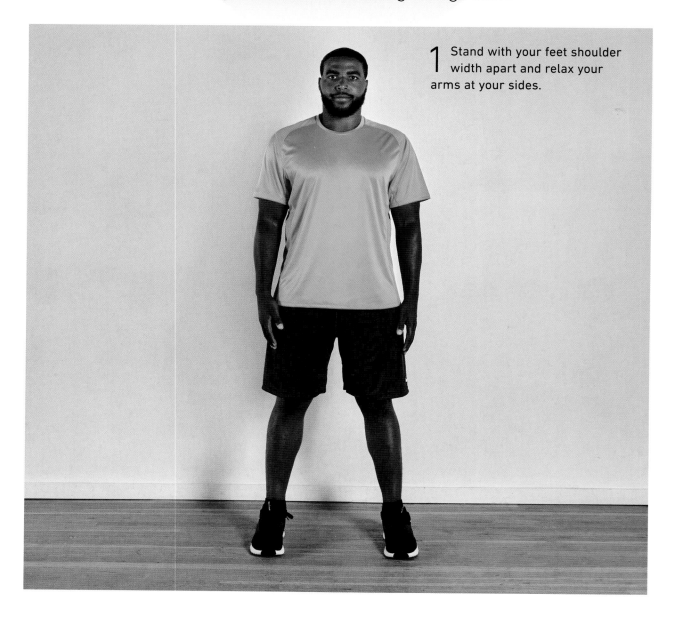

1 Stand with your feet shoulder width apart and relax your arms at your sides.

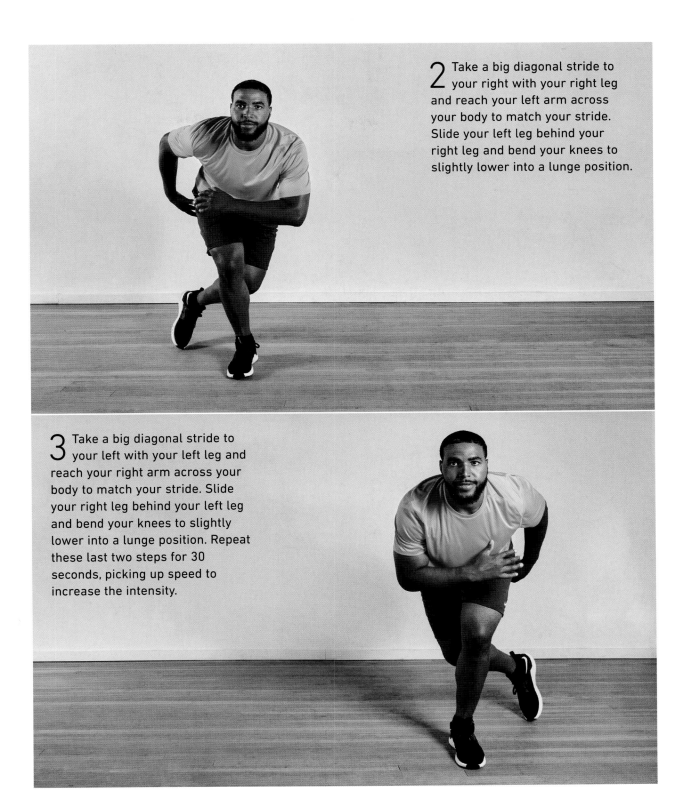

2 Take a big diagonal stride to your right with your right leg and reach your left arm across your body to match your stride. Slide your left leg behind your right leg and bend your knees to slightly lower into a lunge position.

3 Take a big diagonal stride to your left with your left leg and reach your right arm across your body to match your stride. Slide your right leg behind your left leg and bend your knees to slightly lower into a lunge position. Repeat these last two steps for 30 seconds, picking up speed to increase the intensity.

// SPEED SKATING //

VARIATIONS

These modifications remove the speed and complexity.
The options are slower, seated, or without a diagonal pattern.

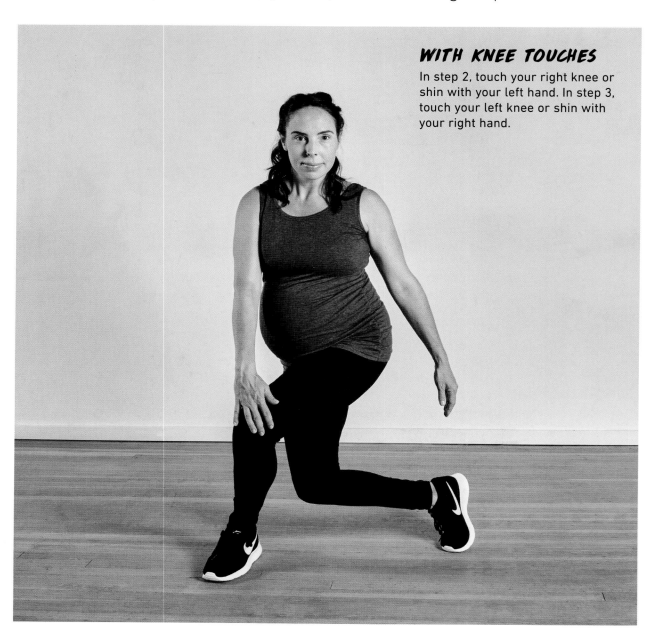

WITH KNEE TOUCHES

In step 2, touch your right knee or shin with your left hand. In step 3, touch your left knee or shin with your right hand.

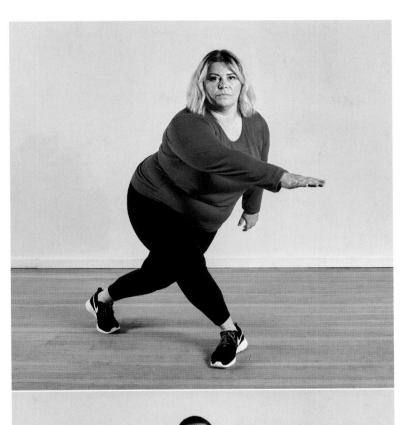

WITH LESS INTENSITY

In steps 2 and 3, perform the movements with little to no bend, a slower tempo, and less impact.

SEATED

1. Sit on the edge of the seat of a chair and place your feet flat on the floor. Relax your arms at your sides.

2. Reach your right arm across your body and extend your left arm backward. (You can also cross your right leg in front of your left leg.)

3. Reach your left arm across your body and extend your right arm backward. (You can also cross your left leg in front of your right leg.) Repeat these last two steps for 30 seconds, picking up speed to increase the intensity.

HIGH KNEES

Performing this exercise will definitely elevate your heart rate and add some coordination-building moves to your routine. These movements will improve your cardiovascular system while primarily engaging your core and quadriceps simultaneously.

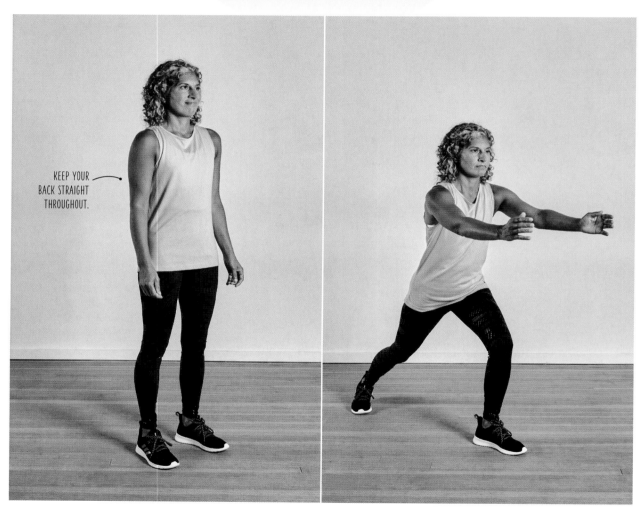

KEEP YOUR
BACK STRAIGHT
THROUGHOUT.

1 Stand with your feet shoulder width apart and relax your arms at your sides.

2 Extend your right leg backward and place the ball of your right foot flat on the floor. Extend your arms until parallel with the floor.

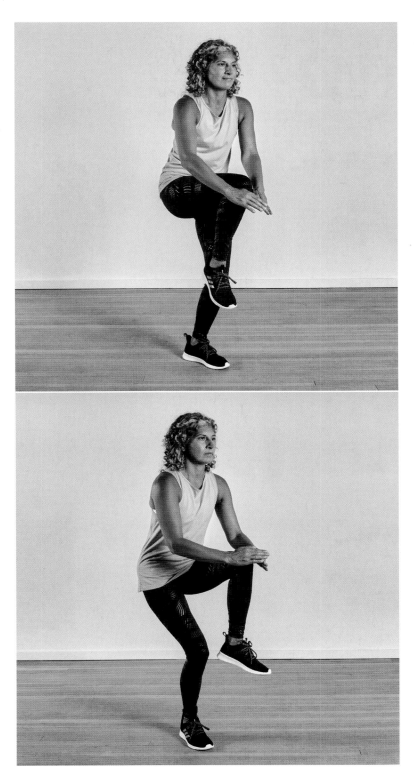

3 Lift your right knee to form a 90-degree angle with your right leg. Lower your arms to touch your right knee with your hands. Pause, then lower your right leg to the floor and extend your arms forward.

4 Lift your left knee to form a 90-degree angle with your left leg. Lower your arms to touch your left knee with your hands. Pause, then lower your left leg to the floor and extend your arms forward. Repeat these last two steps for 30 seconds.

// HIGH KNEES //

VARIATIONS

You can perform this exercise slowly, seated, or with wall support for balance while still elevating your heart rate.

WITH A WALL

1. Stand with your back and heels against a wall. Place your hands flat on the wall and about 1 foot away from your body.

2. Bend your left knee and slowly lift your left knee to form a 90-degree angle with your left leg. Hold this position for 1 second, then return your left leg to the wall.

3. Bend your right knee and slowly lift your right knee to form a 90-degree angle with your right leg. Hold this position for 1 second, then return your right leg to the wall. Repeat these last two steps for 30 seconds.

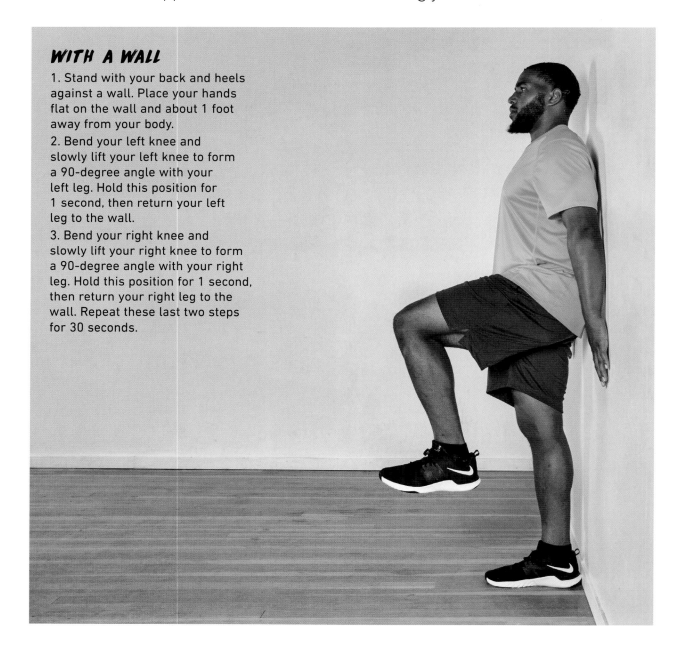

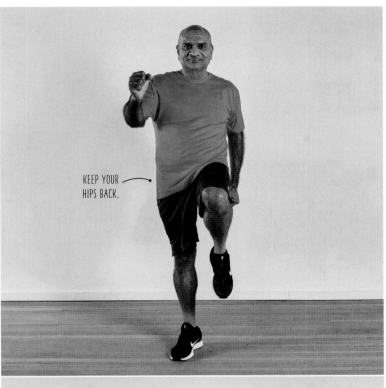

KEEP YOUR HIPS BACK.

MODIFIED MARCHING

1. Stand with your feet shoulder width apart and relax your arms at your sides.

2. Bend your left knee to slowly lift your left leg to form a 90-degree angle with your left leg. Extend your right arm forward in tandem with your left leg. Hold this position for 1 second, then lower your left leg to the floor and lower your right arm to your side.

3. Bend your right knee to slowly lift your right leg to form a 90-degree angle with your right leg. Extend your left arm forward in tandem with your right leg. Hold this position for 1 second, then lower your right leg to the floor and lower your left arm to your side. Repeat these last two steps for 30 seconds.

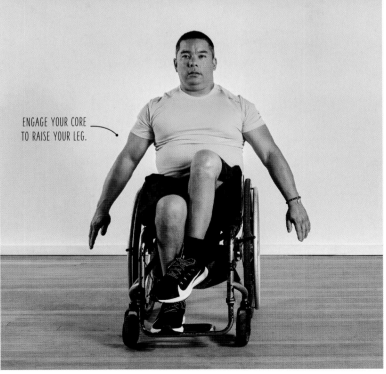

ENGAGE YOUR CORE TO RAISE YOUR LEG.

SEATED

1. Sit in a chair and place your feet flat on the floor. Relax your arms at your sides.

2. Slowly lift your left knee toward your chest. Hold this position for 1 second, then lower your left leg to the floor.

3. Slowly lift your right knee toward your chest. Hold this position for 1 second, then lower your right leg to the floor. Repeat these last two steps for 30 seconds.

GLUTE & LEG EXTENSION

If you're looking to work the backside of your lower body without the compounding demands other exercises place on the body, this extension is an entry-level way to build strength without becoming vulnerable to injury.

1 Place your hands, knees, and the toes of your feet flat on the floor.

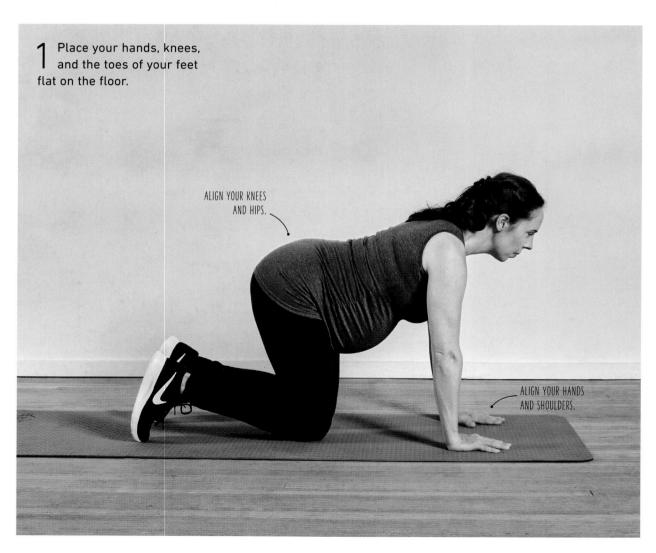

ALIGN YOUR KNEES AND HIPS.

ALIGN YOUR HANDS AND SHOULDERS.

2 Extend your right leg backward until parallel with the floor.

ENGAGE YOUR GLUTES TO RAISE YOUR LEG.

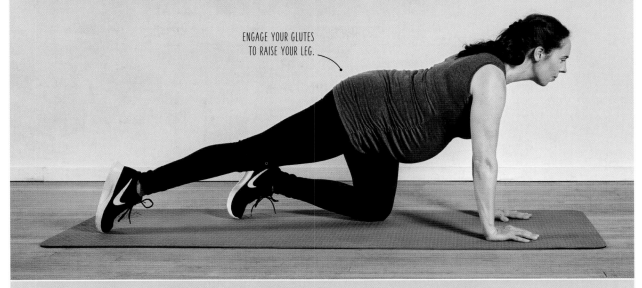

3 Lift your right leg toward the ceiling until your right knee and right shoulder align. Pause, then lower your right leg to the floor. Repeat this step 8 to 10 times. Repeat these steps with your left leg extended backward and lifted.

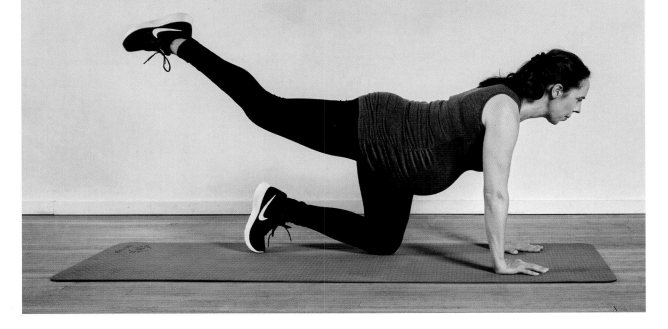

// GLUTE & LEG EXTENSION //

VARIATIONS

If getting down on your knees is a problem,
these modifications offer softer versions with the same results.

WITH A CHAIR

1. Stand behind a chair facing away from you and place your hands on the back of the chair. Step your feet backward about 2 feet.

2. Bend at your waist and extend your right leg backward to form a 45-degree angle with your legs. Pause, then lower your right leg to the floor. Repeat this step 8 to 10 times. Repeat these steps with your left leg extended backward and lifted.

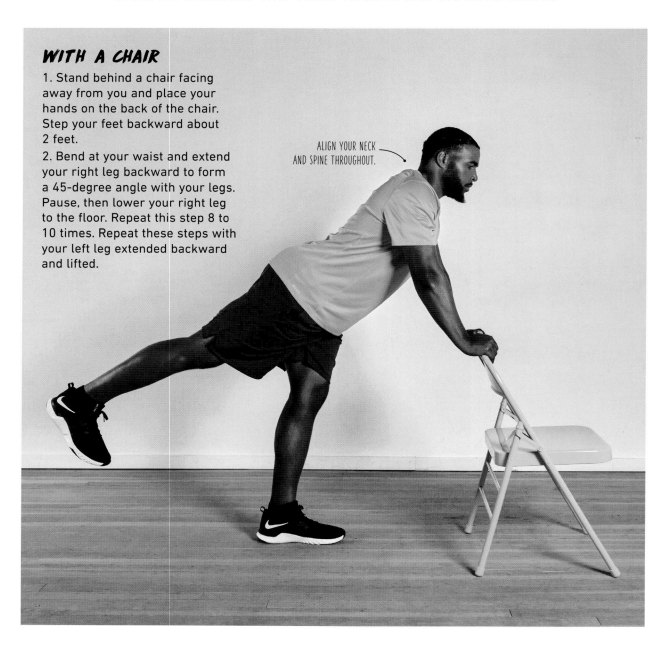

ALIGN YOUR NECK AND SPINE THROUGHOUT.

FLAT ON THE FLOOR

1. Lie flat on your stomach on the floor and place your hands to the outsides of your shoulders.

2. Lift your left leg 1 to 2 feet off the floor. Pause, then lower your left leg to the floor. Repeat this step 8 to 10 times. Repeat these steps with your right leg lifted.

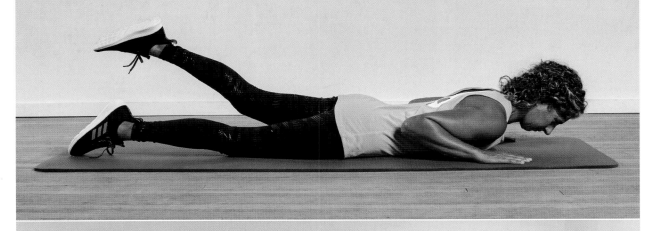

WITH A WALL

1. Stand facing 2 to 3 feet away from a wall and place your hands flat on the wall.

2. Bend at your waist and extend your right leg backward to form a 45-degree angle with your legs. Pause, then lower your right leg to the floor. Repeat this step 8 to 10 times. Repeat these steps with your left leg extended backward and lifted.

ENGAGE YOUR GLUTES TO RAISE YOUR LEG.

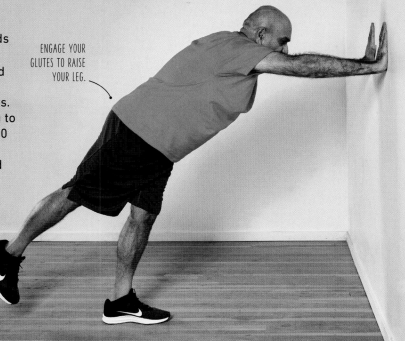

BURPEE

This is a great strength exercise, but it's also a highly effective cardio exercise because it works your shoulders, arms, core, and legs. Plus, the up-and-down motions while raising your arms will always get your heart rate going.

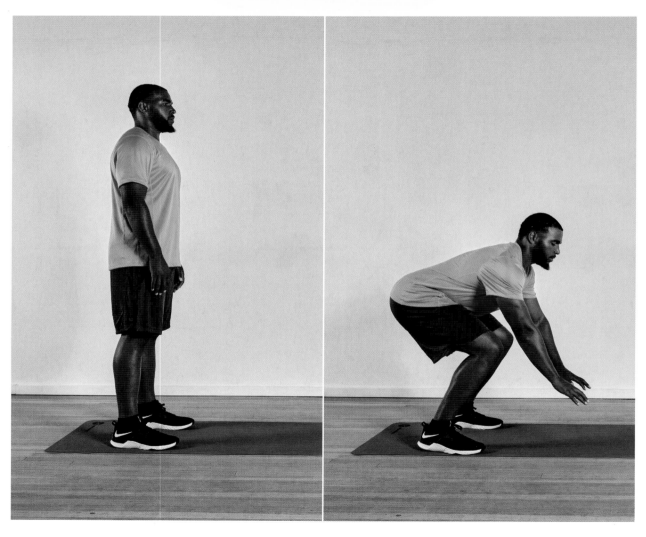

1 Stand with your feet shoulder width apart and relax your arms at your sides.

2 Bend your knees and lower your body into a squat. Reach your hands toward the floor.

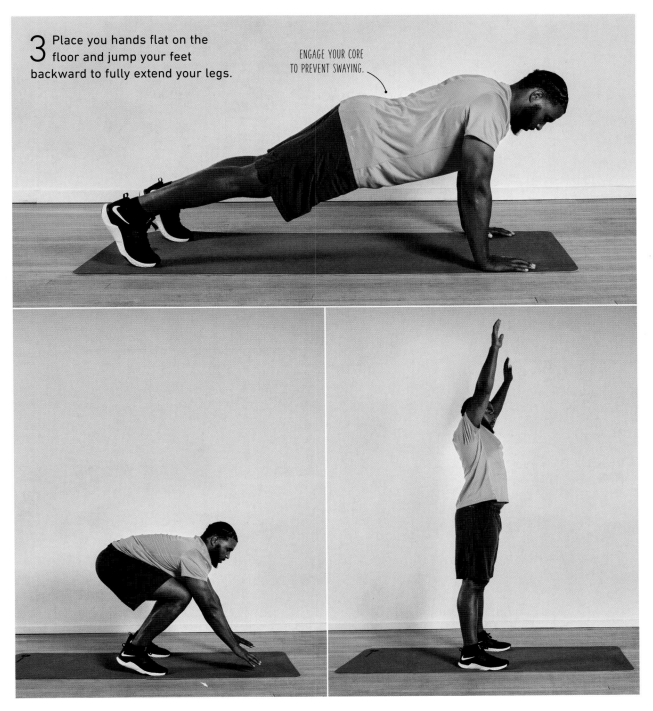

3 Place you hands flat on the floor and jump your feet backward to fully extend your legs.

ENGAGE YOUR CORE TO PREVENT SWAYING.

4 Push through your hands and heels to jump forward into a deep squat.

5 As you begin to stand, extend your arms toward the ceiling. Pause, then lower your arms to your sides. Repeat these last four steps 8 to 10 times.

// BURPEE //
VARIATIONS

Reactions to burpees often include groans. If you perform this exercise with less impact, you might have a different response.

WITH A CHAIR

1. Place the back of a chair against a wall. Stand facing the seat of the chair and relax your arms at your sides.

2. Bend at your waist to place your hands flat on the seat of the chair. Step your feet backward to fully extend your legs.

3. Step toward the chair one foot at a time until you're about 1 foot away from the chair.

4. As you begin to stand, extend your arms toward the ceiling. Pause, then return to your starting position in step 2. Repeat these last three steps 8 to 10 times.

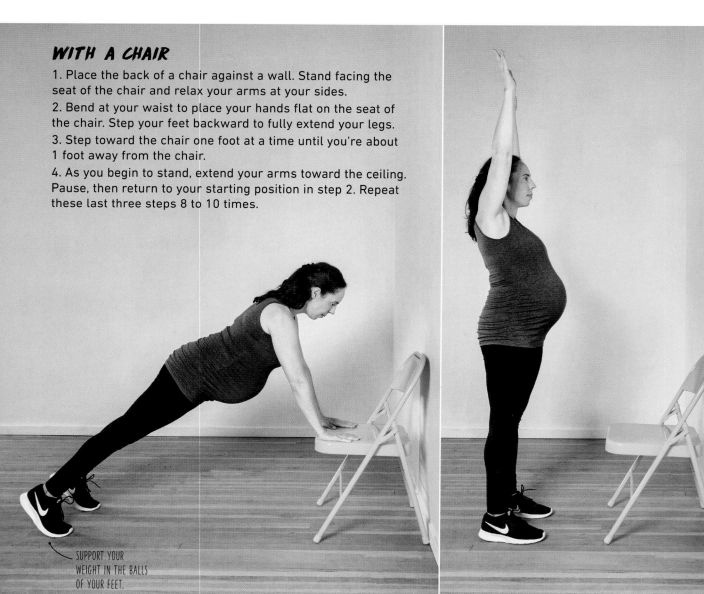

SUPPORT YOUR WEIGHT IN THE BALLS OF YOUR FEET.

WITH LESS INTENSITY

In step 4, step your feet forward one foot at a time. Continue with the remaining steps.

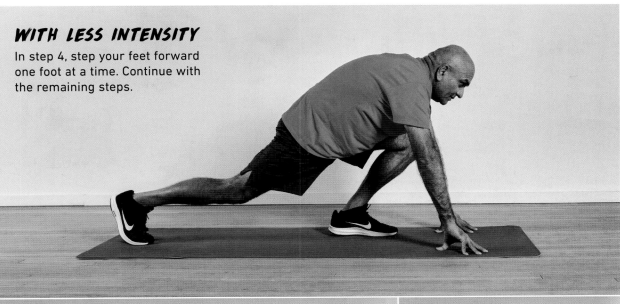

WITH A WALL

1. Stand facing a wall and place your hands flat on the wall. Step backward 2 to 3 feet.

2. Step toward the wall one foot at a time until you're about 1 foot away from the wall.

3. As you begin to stand straight, extend your arms toward the ceiling. Pause, then return to your starting position. Repeat these steps 8 to 10 times.

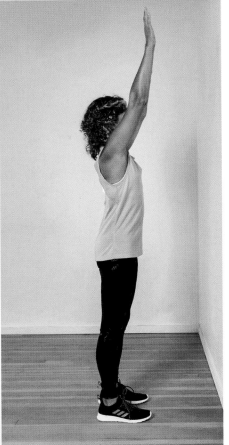

JUMPING JACK

For most of us, jumping jacks are probably the first kind of exercise we ever did as children. They're still effective and intense now that we're adults. If nothing else, they'll certainly increase your heart rate and encourage your stamina.

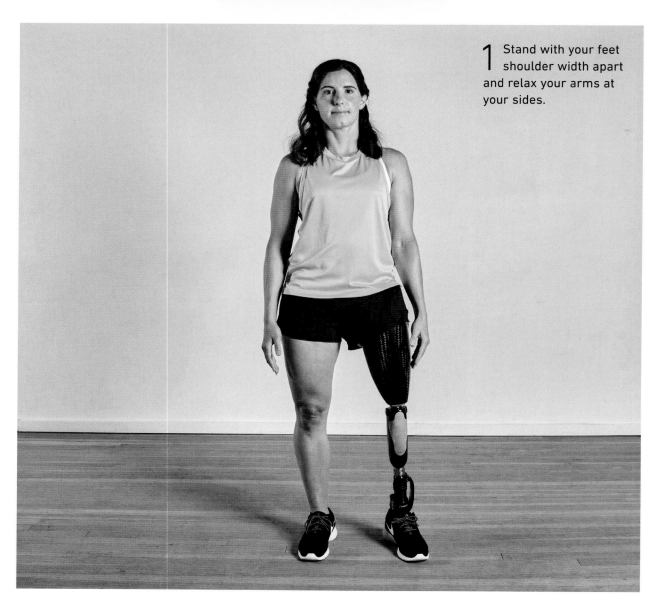

1 Stand with your feet shoulder width apart and relax your arms at your sides.

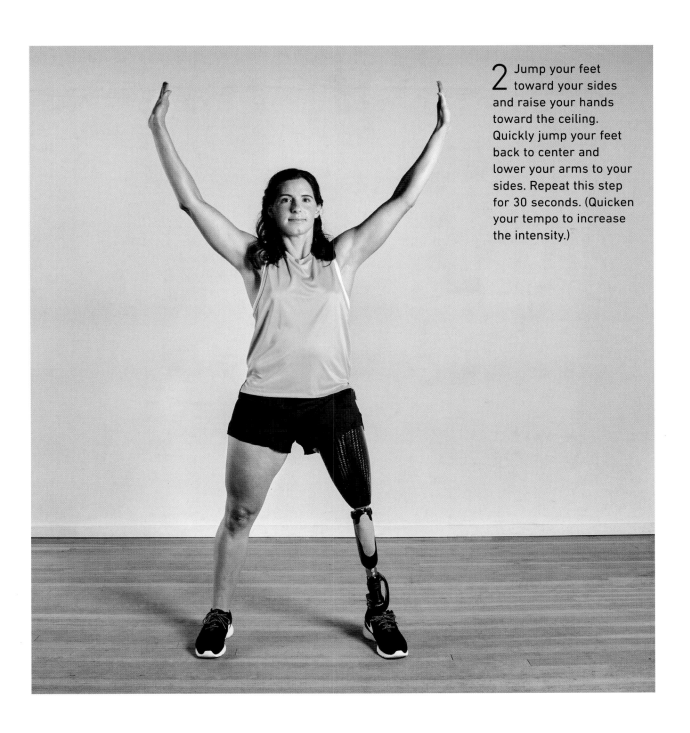

2 Jump your feet toward your sides and raise your hands toward the ceiling. Quickly jump your feet back to center and lower your arms to your sides. Repeat this step for 30 seconds. (Quicken your tempo to increase the intensity.)

VARIATIONS

With these modifications, you can perform a low-impact version, stay seated, or do the movements while lying on the floor.

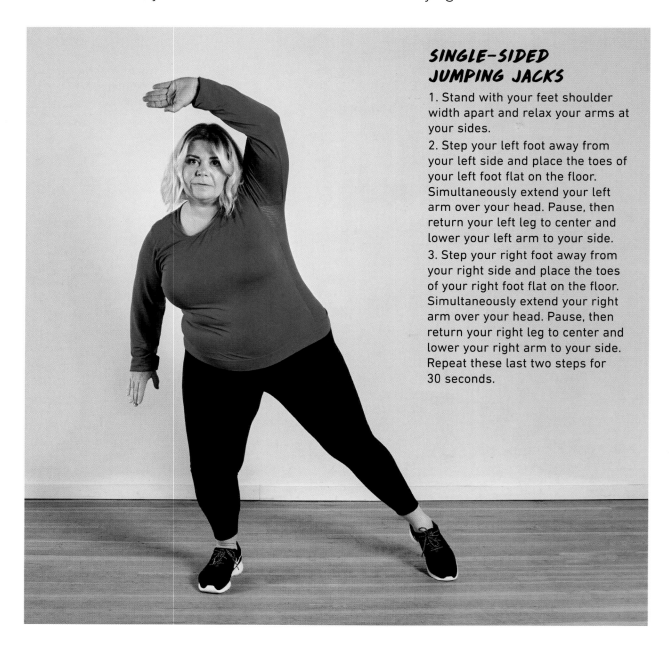

SINGLE-SIDED JUMPING JACKS

1. Stand with your feet shoulder width apart and relax your arms at your sides.

2. Step your left foot away from your left side and place the toes of your left foot flat on the floor. Simultaneously extend your left arm over your head. Pause, then return your left leg to center and lower your left arm to your side.

3. Step your right foot away from your right side and place the toes of your right foot flat on the floor. Simultaneously extend your right arm over your head. Pause, then return your right leg to center and lower your right arm to your side. Repeat these last two steps for 30 seconds.

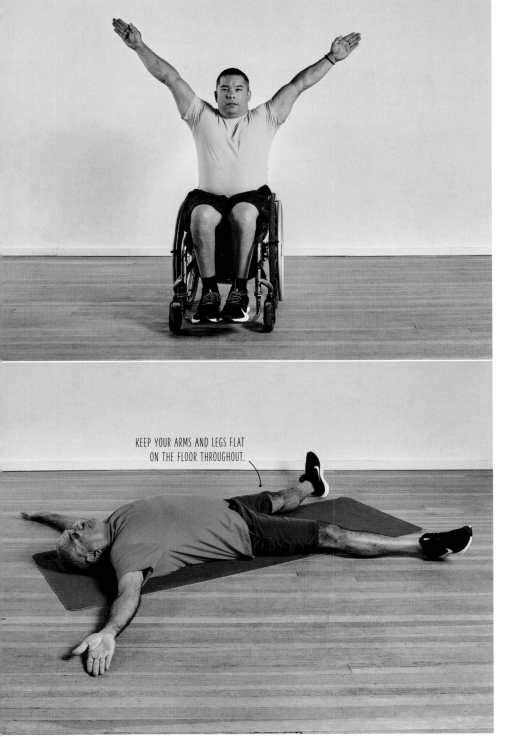

SEATED

1. Sit in a chair and place your feet flat on the floor. Relax your arms at your sides.

2. Extend your arms at 45-degree angles toward the ceiling. (You can also extend your legs to your sides.) Pause, then lower your arms to your sides. Repeat this step for 30 seconds.

ON THE FLOOR

1. Lie on your back on the floor and relax your arms at your sides.

2. Slide your feet toward your sides and extend your arms over your head at 45-degree angles. Pause, then slide your feet back to center and lower your arms to your sides. Repeat this step for 30 seconds.

KEEP YOUR ARMS AND LEGS FLAT ON THE FLOOR THROUGHOUT.

MOUNTAIN CLIMBER

This cardio exercise gives a little spark to your heart rate, but it's also effective at building strength. Because this exercise incorporates your core, hip flexors, and shoulders, you're going to get a full fitness experience with these movements.

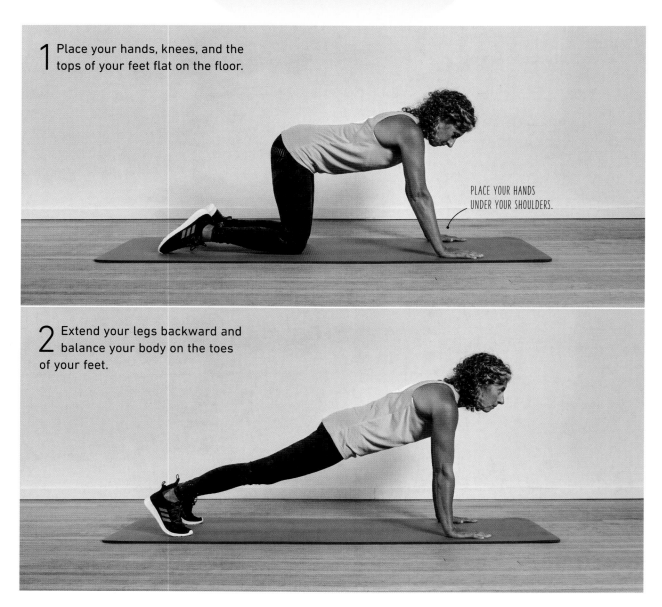

1 Place your hands, knees, and the tops of your feet flat on the floor.

PLACE YOUR HANDS UNDER YOUR SHOULDERS.

2 Extend your legs backward and balance your body on the toes of your feet.

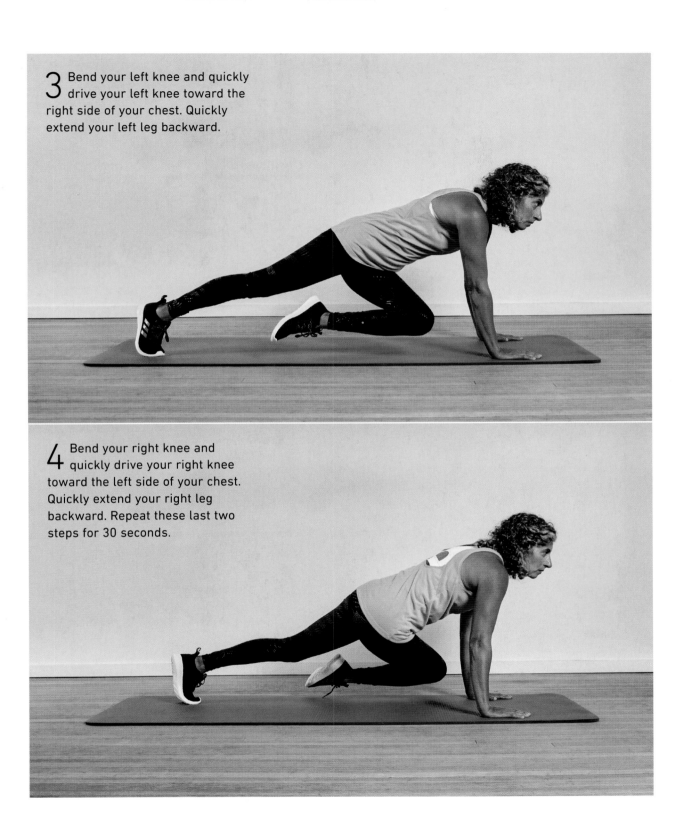

3 Bend your left knee and quickly drive your left knee toward the right side of your chest. Quickly extend your left leg backward.

4 Bend your right knee and quickly drive your right knee toward the left side of your chest. Quickly extend your right leg backward. Repeat these last two steps for 30 seconds.

// MOUNTAIN CLIMBER //

VARIATIONS

Doing this exercise slowly without angling your knee or using a different surface, like a wall or a chair, will make it easier.

WITH LESS INTENSITY

In step 3, bend your right knee to slowly lift your right knee toward the right side of your chest. Slowly extend your right leg backward. Repeat this step for 30 seconds. In step 4, bend your left knee to slowly lift your left knee toward the left side of your chest. Slowly extend your left leg backward. Repeat this step for 30 seconds.

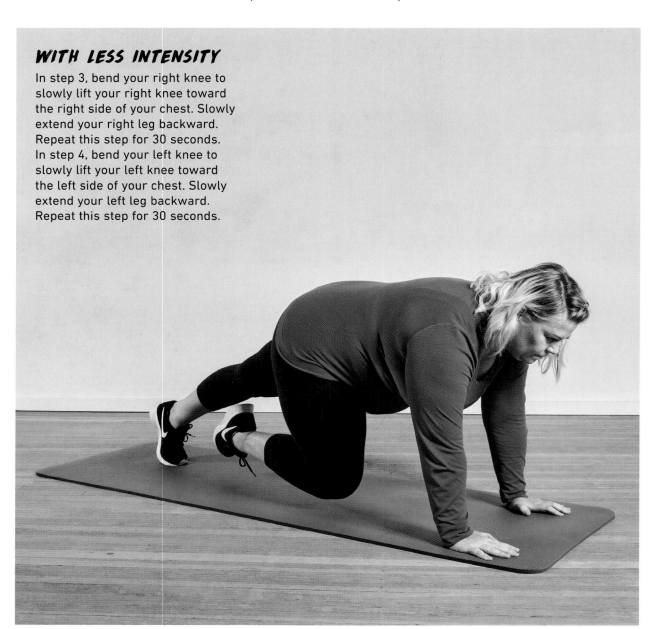

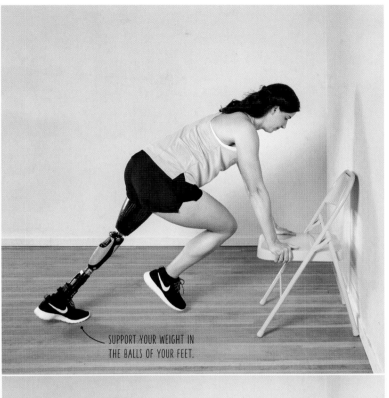

SUPPORT YOUR WEIGHT IN THE BALLS OF YOUR FEET.

WITH A CHAIR

1. Place the back of a chair against a wall. Stand facing the seat of the chair. Relax your arms at your sides.

2. Bend at your waist and place your hands on the sides of the chair. Extend your legs backward.

3. Bend your right knee to slowly lift your right knee toward the left side of your chest. Slowly extend your right leg backward. Repeat this step for 30 seconds.

4. Bend your left knee to slowly lift your left knee toward the right side of your chest. Slowly extend your left leg backward. Repeat this step for 30 seconds.

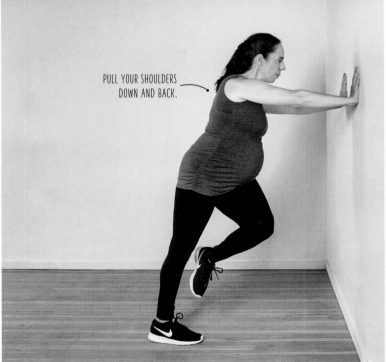

PULL YOUR SHOULDERS DOWN AND BACK.

WITH A WALL

1. Stand facing a wall and place your hands flat on the wall.

2. Step backward 3 to 4 feet and support your weight in the balls of your feet.

3. Bend your left knee and lift your left knee toward the right side of your chest. Return your left leg to the floor. Repeat this step for 30 seconds.

4. Bend your right knee and lift your right knee toward the left side of your chest. Return your right leg to the floor. Repeat this step for 30 seconds.

FAEDRAGH CARPENTER

I was born and raised in Vancouver, British Columbia, and I've always loved taking advantage of the province's beautiful outdoor setting. Specifically, I love taking long walks along our beautiful seawall and breathing in that fresh ocean air! Professionally, I work as a psychiatric nurse and specialize in working with individuals who struggle with mental health and addiction issues. I love the challenges and rewards of my job, and I love being a part of people's journeys in recovery.

I took a real interest in fitness in grade 12 when I joined the community center gym across from my high school. Over the years, I developed a passion for running and I've so far competed in two half-marathons. I love that with fitness and exercise you can set goals for yourself and crush them! And that natural endorphin release through exercise isn't too shabby either! More importantly—and why I was so excited to take part in a book like this—fitness really is for everybody. Regardless of your ability, there are always variations an individual can make to maintain an exercise routine.

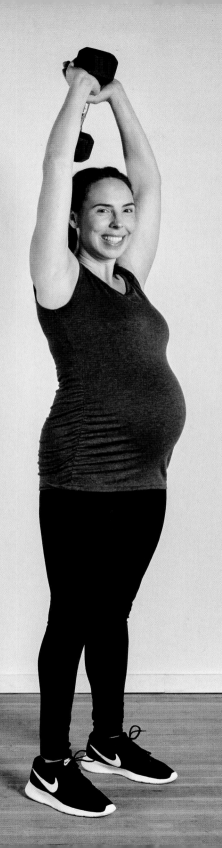

Being almost 9 months pregnant when these photos were taken, I was still able to do lots of the exercises I love—just with some slight modifications. With exercise, there's so much variability and you don't need to have an expensive gym pass to take part. If this is your first time attempting some sort of fitness routine, don't be intimidated. We all have to start somewhere. Start by setting small goals for yourself and build from there. You'll be amazed at how fast you crush them. Good luck!

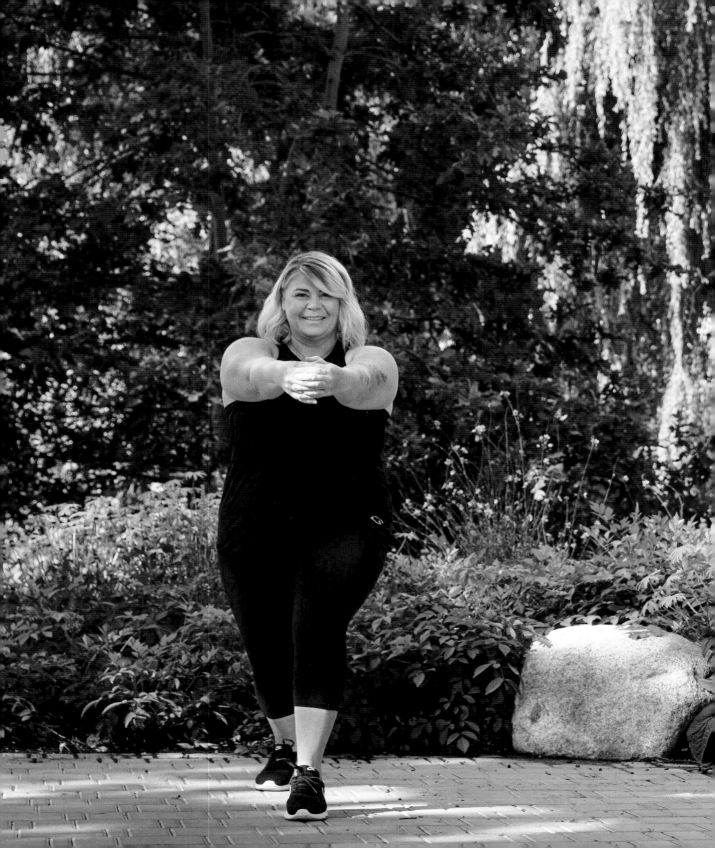

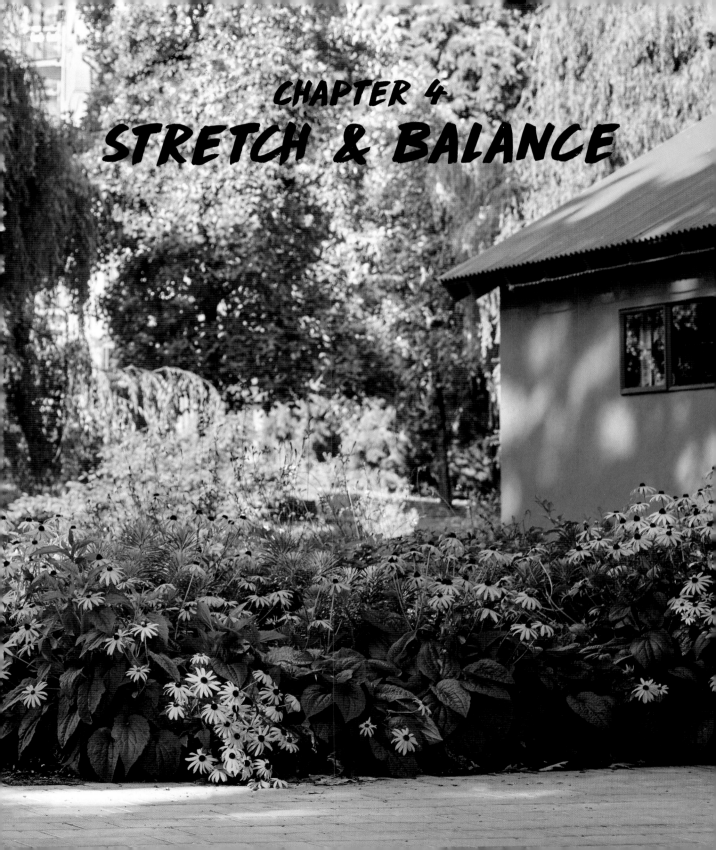

CHAPTER 4
STRETCH & BALANCE

UPPER BACK STRETCH

Having a strong back can help you maintain better posture. Your upper back has many muscles, including the major and minor rhomboids as well as the trapezius. Performing this stretch can help you target and strengthen these muscle groups.

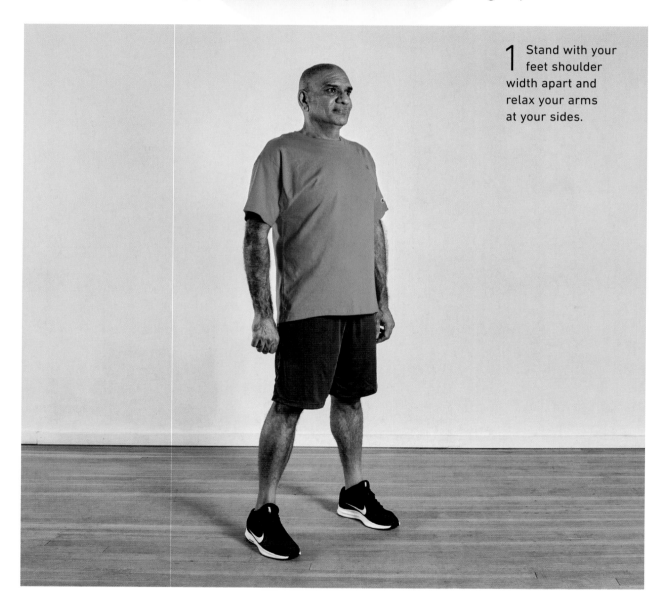

1 Stand with your feet shoulder width apart and relax your arms at your sides.

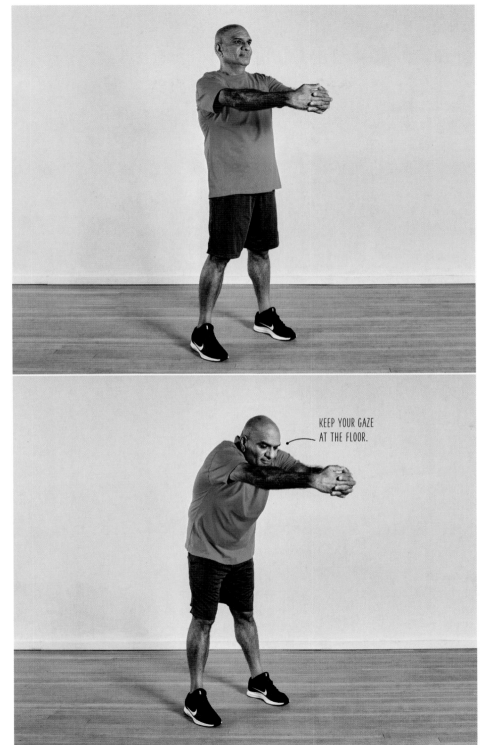

2 Slowly extend your arms forward until parallel with the floor and clasp your hands in front of your chest.

KEEP YOUR GAZE AT THE FLOOR.

3 Lean your head toward your chest and round your upper back. Hold this position for 30 seconds.

// UPPER BACK STRETCH //

VARIATIONS

Because stretching your upper back is important, these seated
and floor options offer similar benefits to the main exercise.

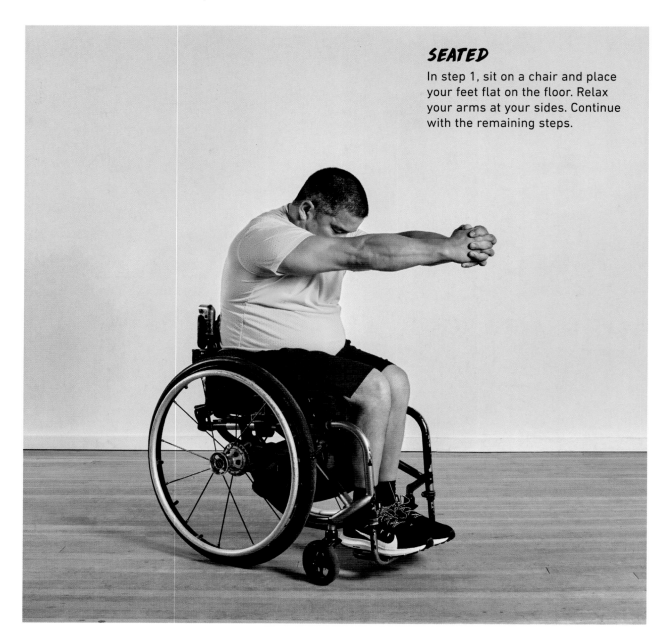

SEATED

In step 1, sit on a chair and place
your feet flat on the floor. Relax
your arms at your sides. Continue
with the remaining steps.

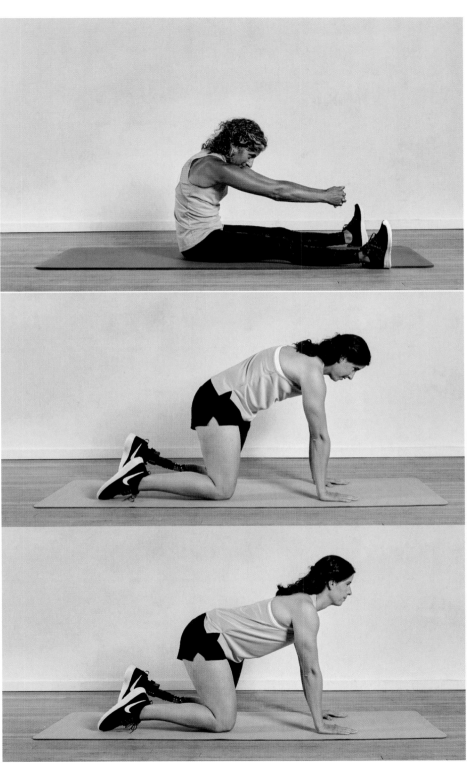

ON THE FLOOR

In step 1, sit on the floor and extend your legs forward. Relax your arms at your sides. Continue with the remaining steps.

CAT-COW

1. Place your hands, knees, and the tops of your feet flat on the floor.

2. Lift your back into a rounded position. Hold this position for 2 to 3 seconds.

3. Lower your hips and lift your gaze until your spine is concave. Hold this position for 2 to 3 seconds. Repeat these last two steps for 30 seconds.

CHEST & PECTORAL STRETCH

People who work at computers tend to roll their shoulders in, compromising their posture. Opening up the chest counters this rounding. Plus, regularly stretching your chest improves your posture and the overall range of motion in your upper body.

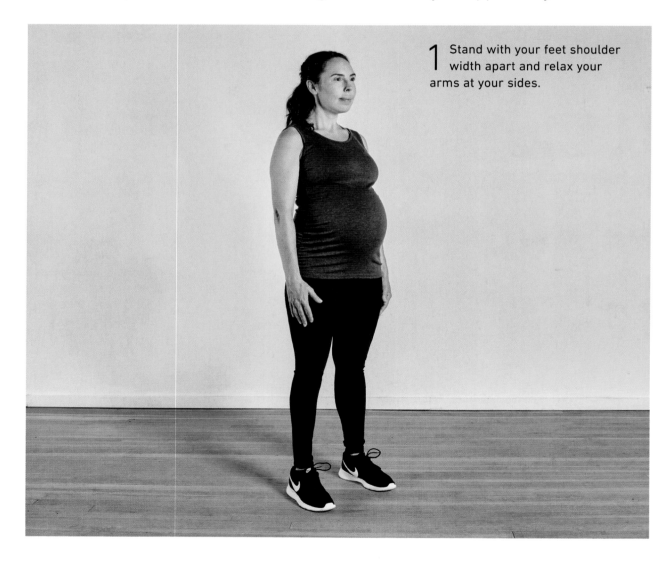

1 Stand with your feet shoulder width apart and relax your arms at your sides.

2 Extend your arms to your sides until aligned with your shoulders. Extend your arms backward as far as possible and push out your chest. Hold this position for 30 seconds.

// CHEST & PECTORAL STRETCH //
VARIATIONS

These modifications mostly give you variety. You might need to try all three to find the one that offers you the deepest stretch.

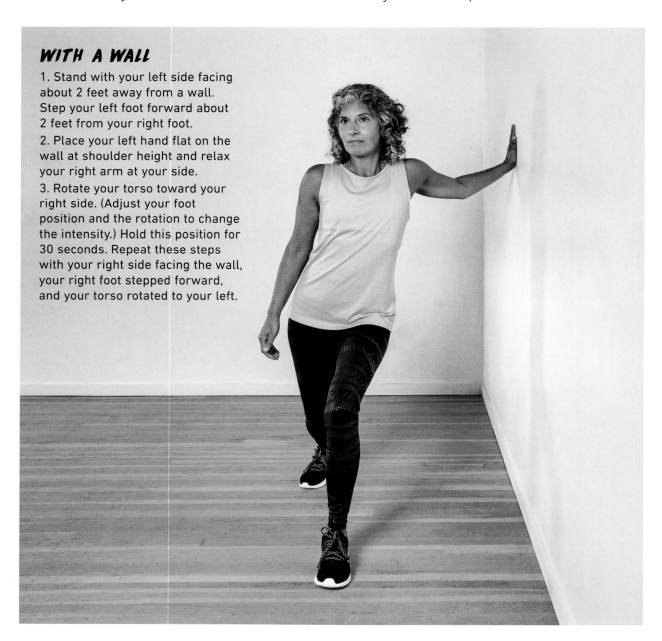

WITH A WALL

1. Stand with your left side facing about 2 feet away from a wall. Step your left foot forward about 2 feet from your right foot.

2. Place your left hand flat on the wall at shoulder height and relax your right arm at your side.

3. Rotate your torso toward your right side. (Adjust your foot position and the rotation to change the intensity.) Hold this position for 30 seconds. Repeat these steps with your right side facing the wall, your right foot stepped forward, and your torso rotated to your left.

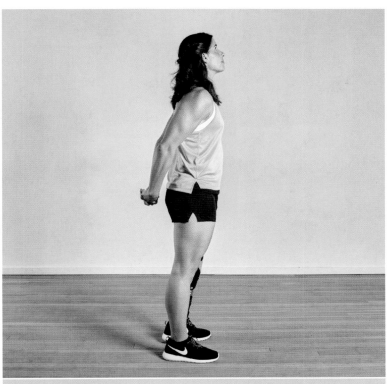

ARMS BEHIND YOU

In step 2, reach your arms behind your lower back and interlock your fingers. Gently squeeze your shoulder blades together and lift your chest toward the ceiling. Hold this position for 30 seconds.

SEATED

1. Sit in a chair and place your feet flat on the floor. Relax your arms at your sides.

2. Place your hands behind your head and interlock your fingers. Slightly push your elbows backward and lift your chest toward the ceiling. Hold this position for 30 seconds.

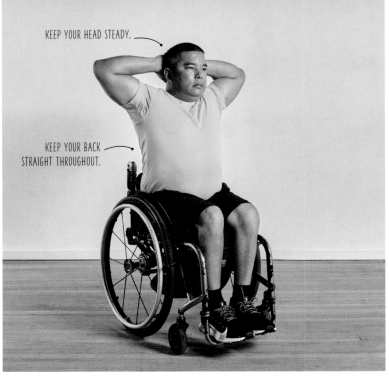

KEEP YOUR HEAD STEADY.

KEEP YOUR BACK STRAIGHT THROUGHOUT.

GLUTE MEDIUS STRETCH

You often hold a lot of tension and tightness in your hips. This glute stretch can provide great relief for these problems. Because tight hips can limit your range of motion, doing this stretch regularly will help with your overall biomechanics.

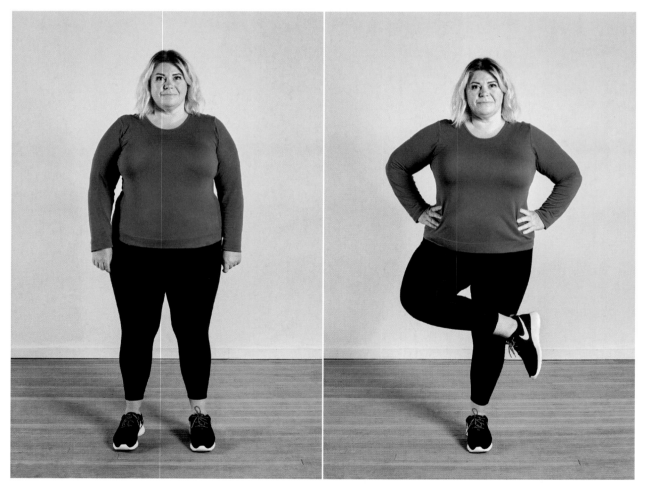

1 Stand with your feet shoulder width apart and relax your arms at your sides.

2 Bend your right knee and place your right ankle on your left knee. Place your hands on your hips.

3 Bend your left knee and slightly lower your body while slightly bending forward from your waist. Hold this position for 30 seconds. Repeat these steps with your left ankle on your right knee.

// GLUTE MEDIUS STRETCH //
VARIATIONS

Everyone has a different level of flexibility. If you find
the main exercise too difficult, try one of these adaptations.

ON THE FLOOR

1. Lie on your back on the floor and place your feet flat on the floor.

2. Bend your left knee to place your left ankle on your right knee.

3. Place your hands behind your right thigh and lift your right leg off the floor to create the stretch. Hold this position for 30 seconds. Repeat these steps with your right ankle on your left knee and with your left leg lifted.

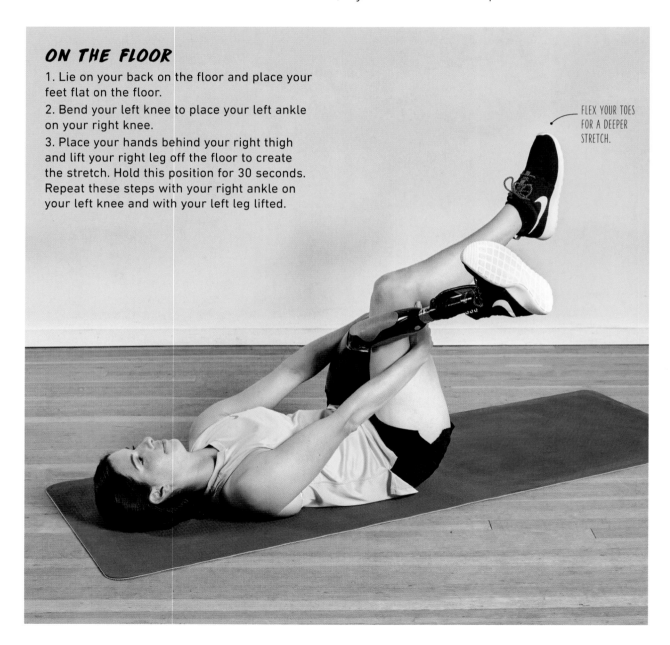

FLEX YOUR TOES FOR A DEEPER STRETCH.

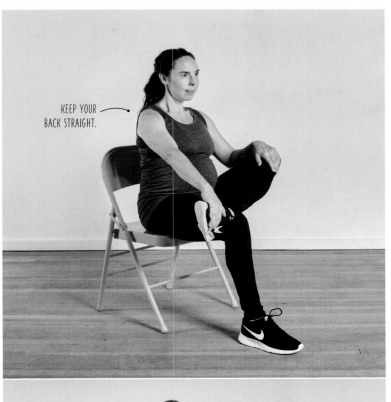

KEEP YOUR BACK STRAIGHT.

SEATED

1. Sit on a chair and place your feet flat on the floor. Relax your arms at your sides.

2. Bend your left knee and place your left ankle on your right knee. Place your left hand on your left knee. (Hold your left foot in your right hand for more stability.) Hold this position for 30 seconds. Repeat these steps with your right ankle on your left knee.

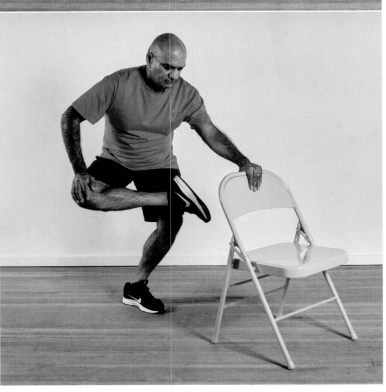

WITH A CHAIR

1. Stand on the right side of a chair with your feet shoulder width apart. Place your left hand on the back of the chair and relax your right arm at your side.

2. Bend your right knee and place your right ankle on your left knee. Place your right hand on your right knee for stability.

3. Bend your left knee and slightly lower your body while slightly bending forward. Hold this position for 30 seconds. Repeat these steps on the left side of the chair with your right hand on the back of the chair and your left ankle on your right knee.

OBLIQUE & LAT STRETCH

You'll feel this stretch between your ribs and pelvis. You'll also notice the impact on your lower back. When stretched regularly, these areas can enjoy fluidity for better range of motion within the torso and more ease within the ribs for breathing.

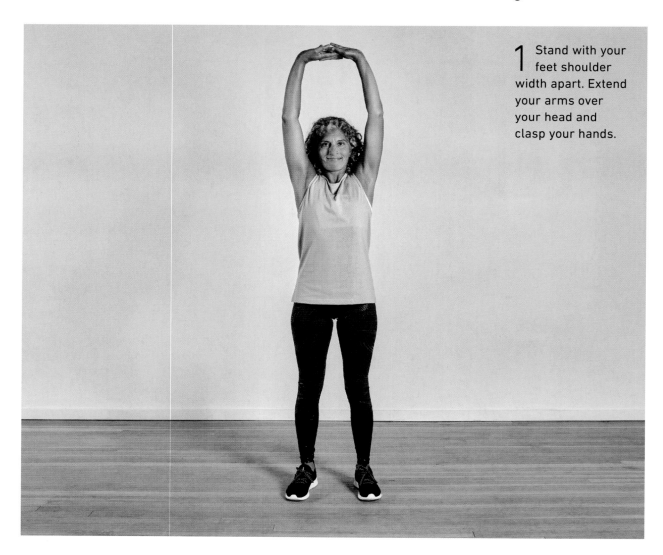

1 Stand with your feet shoulder width apart. Extend your arms over your head and clasp your hands.

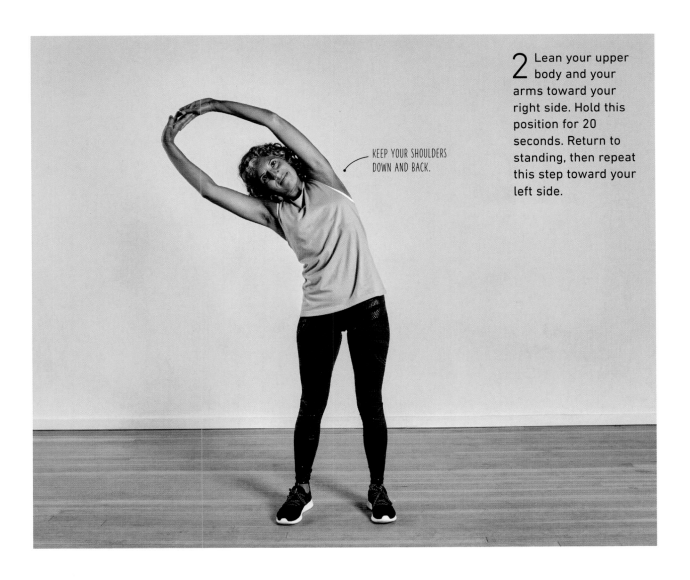

KEEP YOUR SHOULDERS
DOWN AND BACK.

2 Lean your upper body and your arms toward your right side. Hold this position for 20 seconds. Return to standing, then repeat this step toward your left side.

// OBLIQUE & LAT STRETCH //

VARIATIONS

Everyone feels this stretch differently, making execution key.
These options let you deepen the stretch in a way that suits you.

WITH A WALL

1. Stand with your left side facing a wall and your feet shoulder width apart. Relax your arms at your sides.

2. Place your left hand flat on the wall and extend your right arm toward the ceiling.

3. Lean your body and your right arm toward the wall as far as is comfortable. Hold this position for 30 seconds, then return to center. Repeat these steps with your right side facing a wall and your left arm and your body leaning toward the wall.

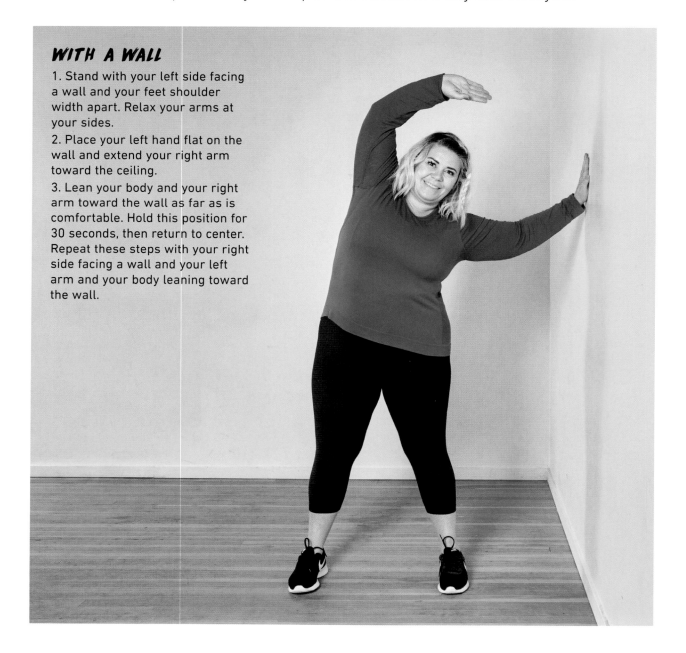

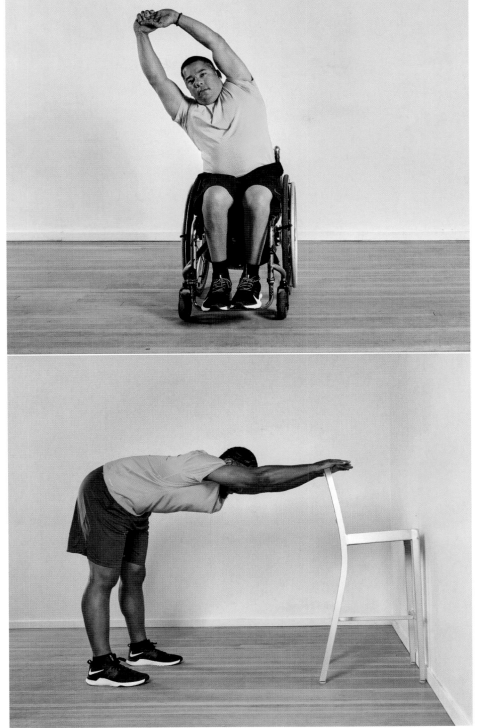

SEATED

In step 1, sit on a chair and place your feet flat on the floor. Raise your arms over your head and clasp your hands. Continue with the remaining step.

WITH A CHAIR

1. Place the seat of a chair flat against a wall. Stand about 1 foot behind the back of the chair and place your hands on the back of the chair.

2. Walk your feet backward until your chest is parallel with the floor. Hold this position for 20 seconds.

HIP FLEXOR STRETCH

Your hip flexors (iliopsoas) play a major role in walking, running, and standing, but they also shorten when you sit for too long. This can compromise your biomechanics, but lengthening your hip flexors is good practice for a sound moving body.

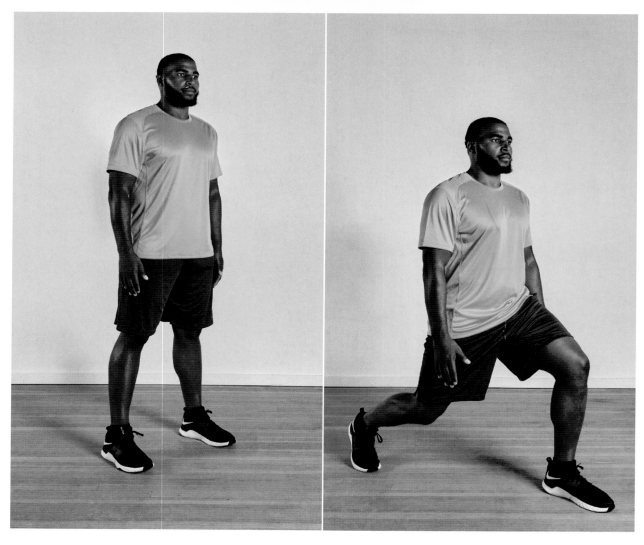

1 Stand with your feet shoulder width apart and relax your arms at your sides.

2 Step your left foot forward 1 to 2 feet and lower your body into a lunge position.

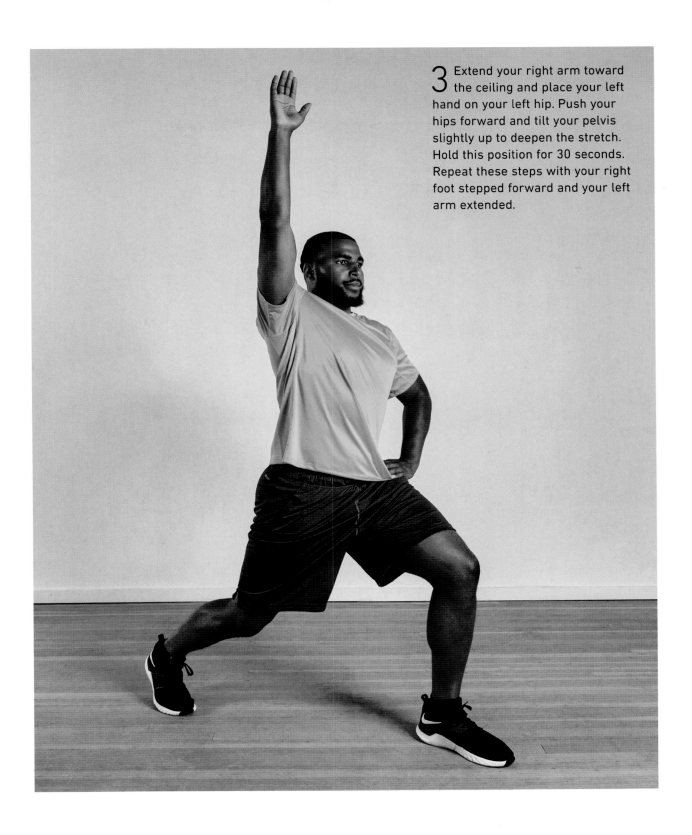

3 Extend your right arm toward the ceiling and place your left hand on your left hip. Push your hips forward and tilt your pelvis slightly up to deepen the stretch. Hold this position for 30 seconds. Repeat these steps with your right foot stepped forward and your left arm extended.

// HIP FLEXOR STRETCH //

VARIATIONS

These options offer a shallower approach as well as sitting
and kneeling modifications if you have any issues with balance.

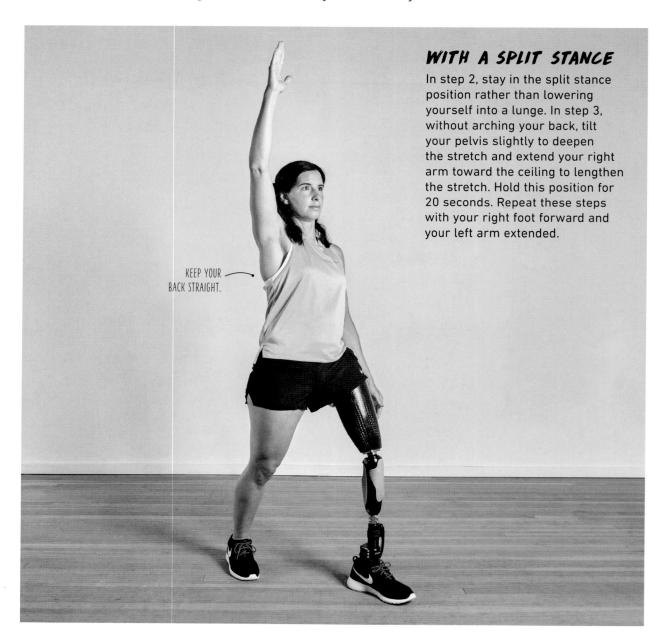

KEEP YOUR
BACK STRAIGHT.

WITH A SPLIT STANCE

In step 2, stay in the split stance
position rather than lowering
yourself into a lunge. In step 3,
without arching your back, tilt
your pelvis slightly to deepen
the stretch and extend your right
arm toward the ceiling to lengthen
the stretch. Hold this position for
20 seconds. Repeat these steps
with your right foot forward and
your left arm extended.

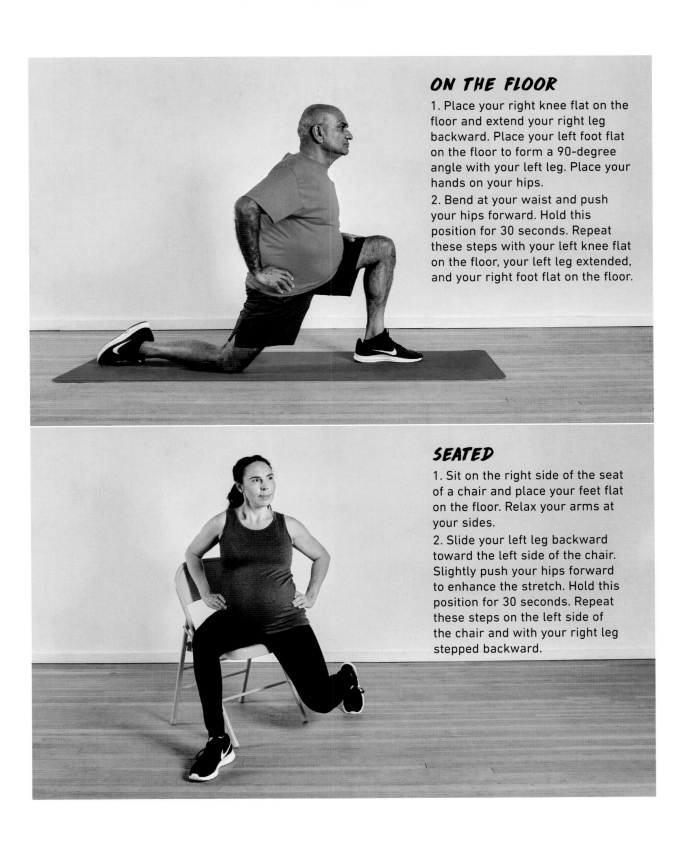

ON THE FLOOR

1. Place your right knee flat on the floor and extend your right leg backward. Place your left foot flat on the floor to form a 90-degree angle with your left leg. Place your hands on your hips.

2. Bend at your waist and push your hips forward. Hold this position for 30 seconds. Repeat these steps with your left knee flat on the floor, your left leg extended, and your right foot flat on the floor.

SEATED

1. Sit on the right side of the seat of a chair and place your feet flat on the floor. Relax your arms at your sides.

2. Slide your left leg backward toward the left side of the chair. Slightly push your hips forward to enhance the stretch. Hold this position for 30 seconds. Repeat these steps on the left side of the chair and with your right leg stepped backward.

CALF STRETCH

Our calves take constant hits from walking, running, climbing stairs, or just standing. They get tight! Whether you've worked out or not, stretching your calves is something you should do often. Your everyday routines will thank you!

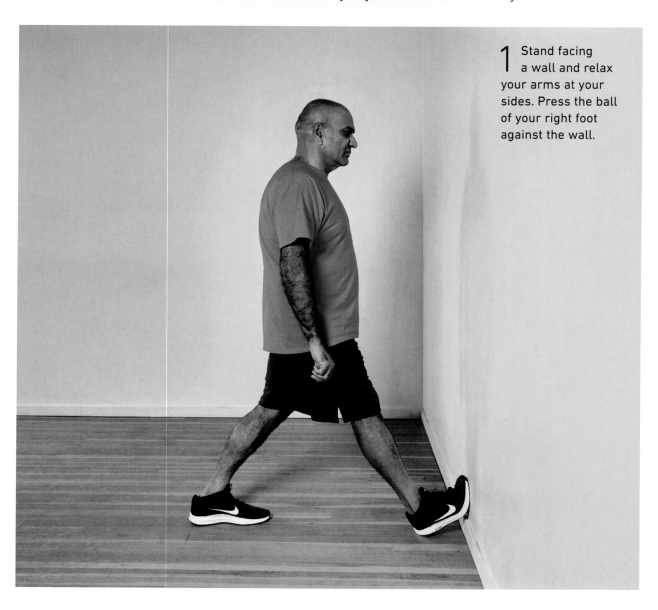

1 Stand facing a wall and relax your arms at your sides. Press the ball of your right foot against the wall.

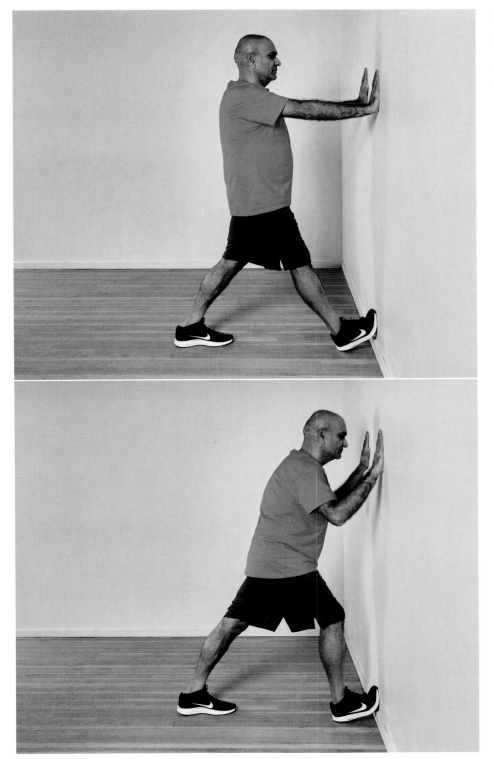

2 Place your hands flat on the wall. (Adjust where you stand to be in a more comfortable position.)

3 Bend your elbows and lean your body toward the wall. Hold this position for 30 seconds. Repeat these steps with the ball of your left foot pressed against the wall.

// CALF STRETCH //
VARIATIONS

These modifications offer a freestanding version as well as seated and wall-assisted options to help if balance is an issue.

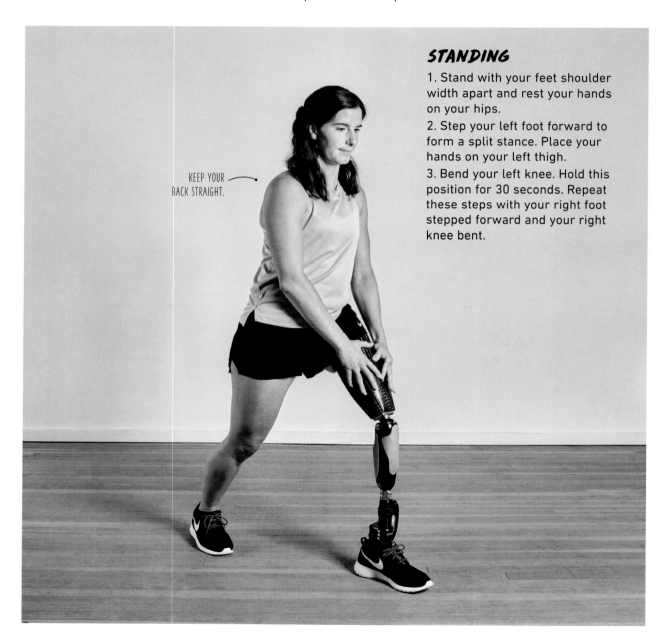

KEEP YOUR
BACK STRAIGHT.

STANDING

1. Stand with your feet shoulder width apart and rest your hands on your hips.
2. Step your left foot forward to form a split stance. Place your hands on your left thigh.
3. Bend your left knee. Hold this position for 30 seconds. Repeat these steps with your right foot stepped forward and your right knee bent.

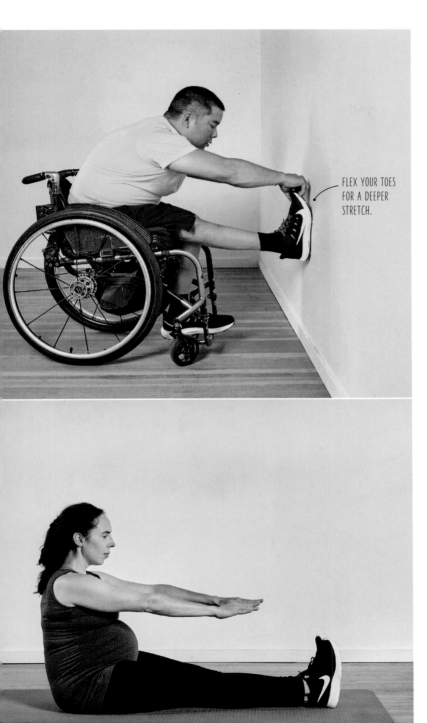

FLEX YOUR TOES FOR A DEEPER STRETCH.

SEATED & WITH A WALL

1. Sit in a chair facing a wall and place your feet flat on the floor. Relax your arms at your sides.

2. Extend your right leg forward and place your right foot flat against the wall. (Adjust the chair's placement as needed.)

3. Bend at your waist to extend your right arm forward to grab your right foot with your right hand. Hold this position for 30 seconds. Repeat these steps with your left leg and left arm.

ON THE FLOOR

1. Sit on the floor and extend your arms and legs forward.

2. Flex your feet toward your body until you feel tension in your calves. Hold this position for 2 to 3 seconds. Unflex your feet, then repeat this step 8 to 10 times.

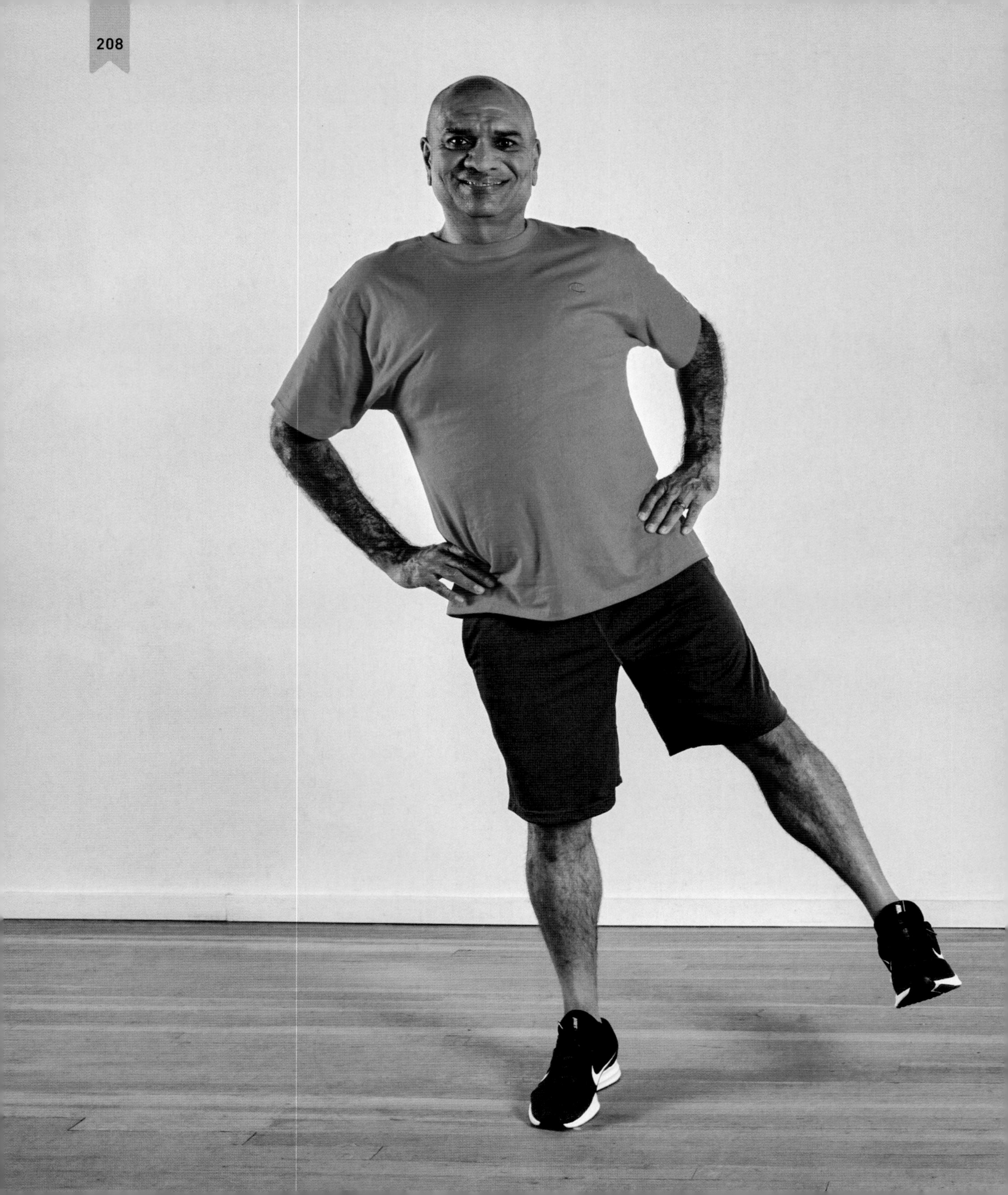

TAZ VISRAM

I'm still evolving and I hope that never changes! My family says I'm a big kid and I wouldn't want it any other way. I was born in Tanzania but moved to Canada when I was 13. I lived in Toronto until I moved to Vancouver in 2013 (which is seriously the best place on Earth—and also the center of the universe because my wife lives here!). I have a degree in technical engineering, so I like complex problems and finding solutions to them. I love good food—eating it and cooking it. I lose stuff a lot, but it's all good: My wife helps me find whatever it is because she's the one who hides it in the first place.

I was once a big guy. I was diabetic and out of shape. Any type of exercise was hard. It still is—but not in the same way. Now it's a good "hard." Challenging myself physically to do more with my personal trainer or to improve my form or to try new activities I haven't done before is rewarding. I'm amazed at what my body can do, how I've improved, and how much better life is. In fact, I believe I'm more fit and active now than I was in my teens and early twenties (even while playing football in high school). Exercise or activity of any sort needs to be a part of my life—of every life. I feel better mentally and physically because of it and because of all the inspiring people I meet along the way.

I love cycling—like, really, really, really love cycling. I cycled when I was in Toronto, but the move to Vancouver changed my life because I was able to cycle year-round. It was a game-changer! I've completed five Ride to Conquer Cancer events (with one being virtual because of COVID-19) and I'll continue to ride as long as I'm physically able. Adding other activities, physical therapy sessions, and yoga has only helped me get stronger, which makes me an even better cyclist. You know, I used to hate hills. Now I embrace them: I look forward to them and I chase them.

I recently conquered riding my bike up Cypress Mountain! It was hard, but I didn't give up. In the past, I would have stopped or given up. I continued on and reached the top. Total elevation on that ride was close to 1,400 meters! Life is amazing, and without an active lifestyle, I wouldn't have been able to complete this ride and it wouldn't have been as great!

HAMSTRING STRETCH

Hamstrings help you walk, bend your knees, and tilt your pelvis.
This stretch can help increase your flexibility, strengthen the
range of motion in your hips, and reduce low back pain.
That makes this great for performing at the end of a workout.

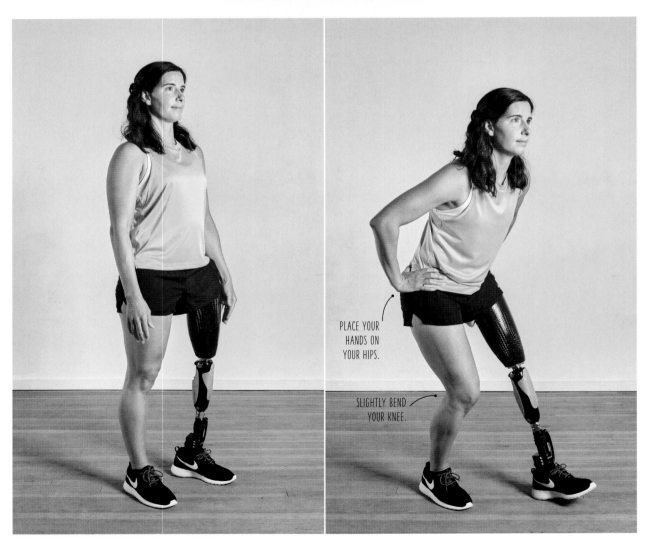

PLACE YOUR
HANDS ON
YOUR HIPS.

SLIGHTLY BEND
YOUR KNEE.

1 Stand with your feet shoulder width apart and relax your arms at your sides.

2 Step your left foot forward and balance your left leg on your heel. Place your hands on your hips.

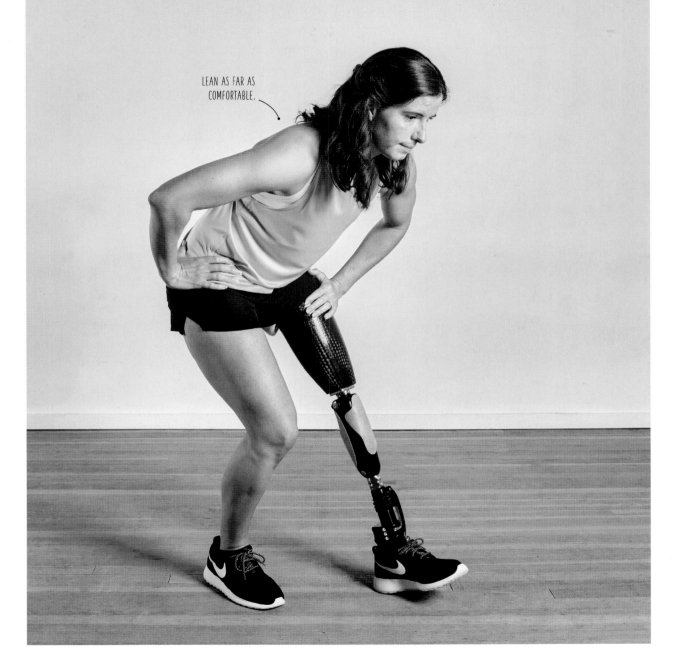

3 Bend at your waist until you feel a stretch in the back of your upper left leg. Hold this position for 30 seconds, then return to standing. Repeat these last two steps with your right foot stepped forward.

LEAN AS FAR AS COMFORTABLE.

// HAMSTRING STRETCH //
VARIATIONS

Try one of these options—seated on a chair or on the floor—
to deepen the stretch without thinking about balance.

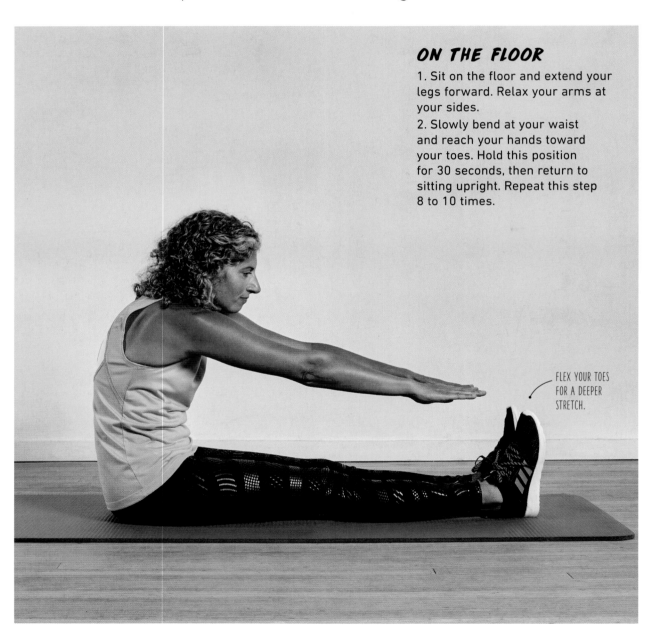

ON THE FLOOR

1. Sit on the floor and extend your legs forward. Relax your arms at your sides.
2. Slowly bend at your waist and reach your hands toward your toes. Hold this position for 30 seconds, then return to sitting upright. Repeat this step 8 to 10 times.

FLEX YOUR TOES FOR A DEEPER STRETCH.

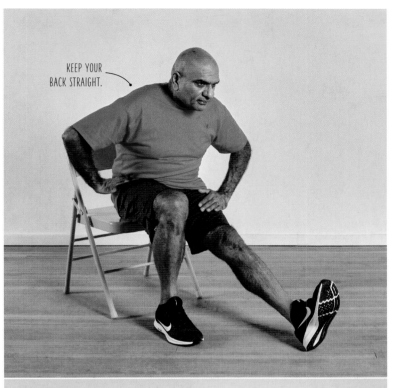

KEEP YOUR
BACK STRAIGHT.

SEATED

1. Sit on the edge of the seat of a chair and place your feet flat on the floor. Place your hands on your hips.

2. Extend your left leg forward and balance your left leg on your left heel.

3. Bend at your waist until you can feel a stretch in the back of your upper left leg. Hold this position for 30 seconds, then return to sitting upright. Repeat these steps with your right foot stepped forward.

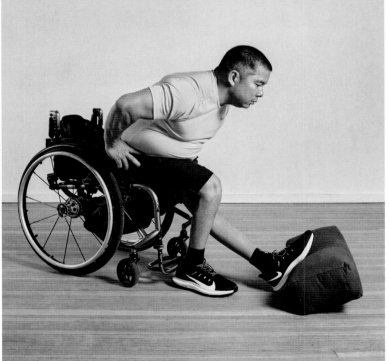

SEATED WITH A BOLSTER

1. Sit on the edge of the seat of a chair and place your feet flat on the floor. Relax your arms at your sides.

2. Extend your left leg forward and place your left foot on a bolster. Place your hands on your hips.

3. Bend at your waist until you can feel a stretch in the back of your upper left leg. Hold this position for 30 seconds, then return to sitting upright. Repeat these steps with your right foot stepped forward.

SHOULDER STRETCH

Shoulders are a common area for injury, but regularly stretching can strengthen shoulder muscles. Plus, stretches can help with posture and biomechanics by activating the three heads of the shoulder muscles: the posterior, medial, and anterior deltoids.

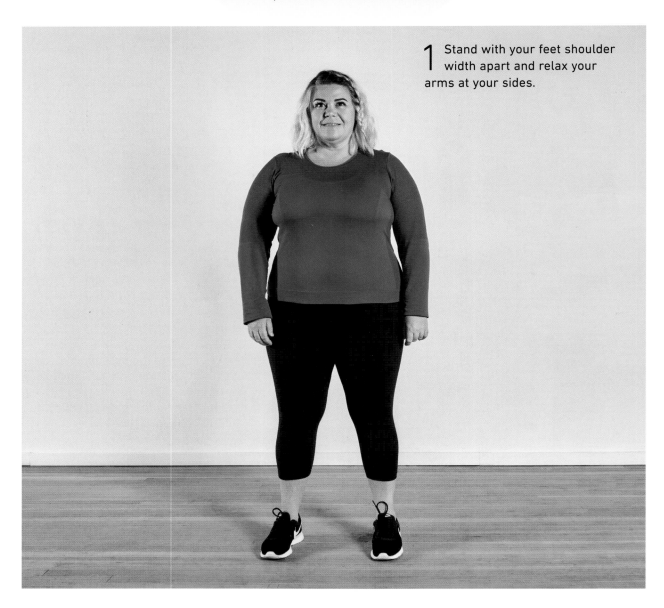

1 Stand with your feet shoulder width apart and relax your arms at your sides.

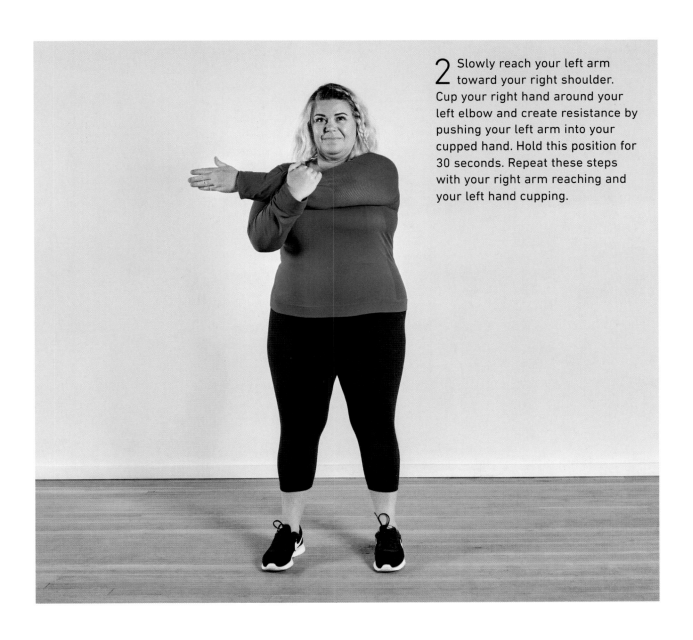

2 Slowly reach your left arm toward your right shoulder. Cup your right hand around your left elbow and create resistance by pushing your left arm into your cupped hand. Hold this position for 30 seconds. Repeat these steps with your right arm reaching and your left hand cupping.

// SHOULDER STRETCH //
VARIATIONS

Try these variations to see which one is best for you.
If standing is challenging, check out the seated option.

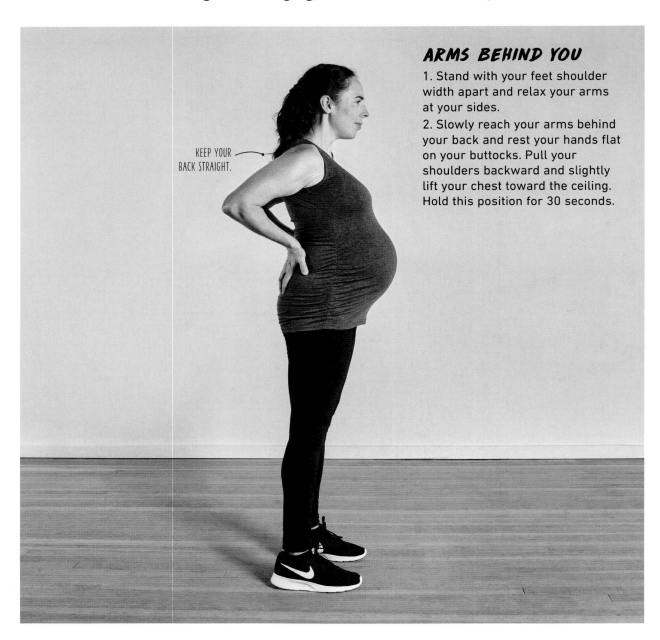

KEEP YOUR
BACK STRAIGHT.

ARMS BEHIND YOU

1. Stand with your feet shoulder width apart and relax your arms at your sides.

2. Slowly reach your arms behind your back and rest your hands flat on your buttocks. Pull your shoulders backward and slightly lift your chest toward the ceiling. Hold this position for 30 seconds.

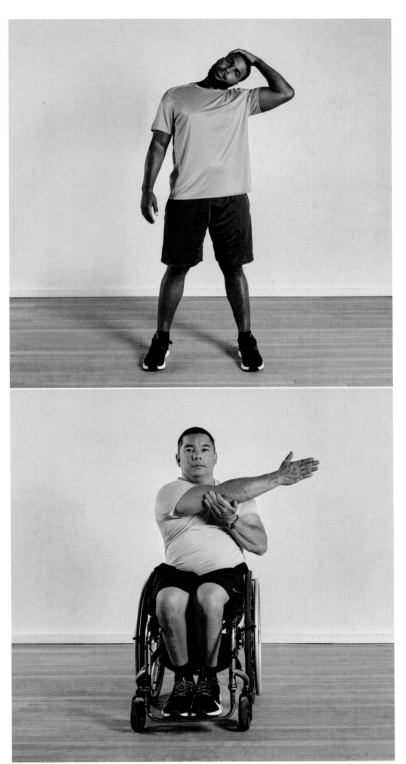

WITH HEAD PULLS

1. Stand with your feet shoulder width apart and relax your arms at your sides.

2. Lean your head toward your left side and drop your right shoulder. Place your left hand on the right side of your face and gently pull to help with the stretch. Hold this position for 30 seconds, then return to your starting position.

3. Lean your head toward your right side and drop your left shoulder. Place your right hand on the left side of your face and gently pull to help with the stretch. Hold this position for 30 seconds.

SEATED

In step 1, sit on a chair and place your feet flat on the floor. Relax your arms at your sides. Continue with the remaining step.

QUAD STRETCH

Your quadriceps are a large group of four muscles at the front of your leg—from above the knee to your hip. Tight quads can cause problems with your knees and hips, but this stretch is a great way to work your quads.

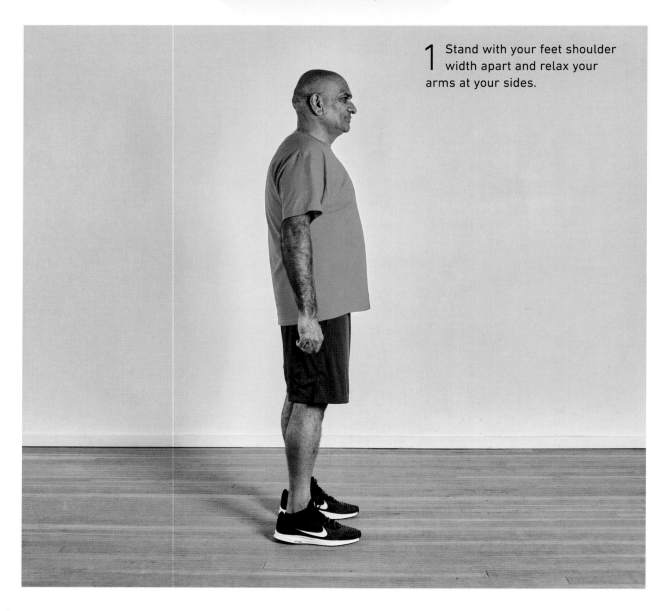

1 Stand with your feet shoulder width apart and relax your arms at your sides.

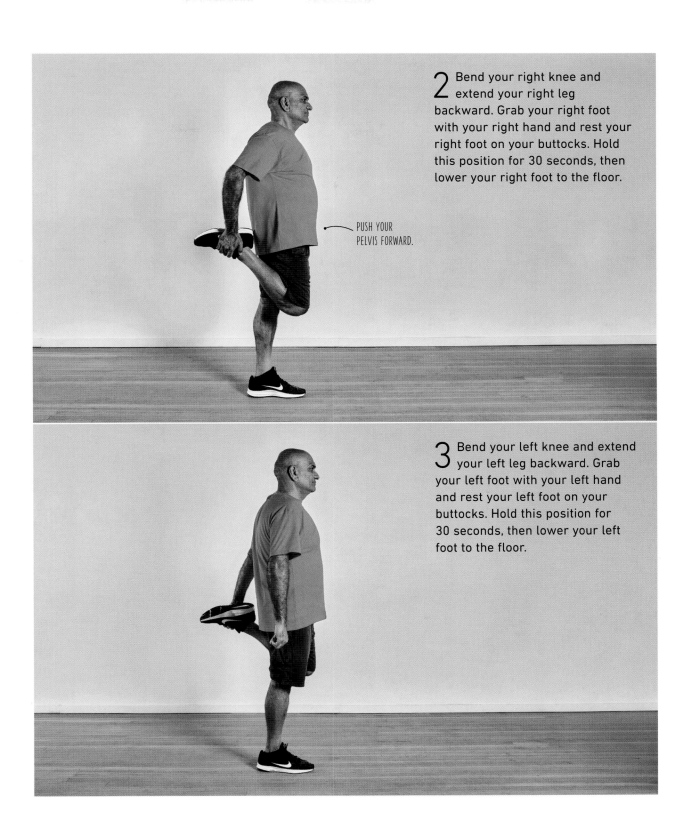

2 Bend your right knee and extend your right leg backward. Grab your right foot with your right hand and rest your right foot on your buttocks. Hold this position for 30 seconds, then lower your right foot to the floor.

PUSH YOUR PELVIS FORWARD.

3 Bend your left knee and extend your left leg backward. Grab your left foot with your left hand and rest your left foot on your buttocks. Hold this position for 30 seconds, then lower your left foot to the floor.

// QUAD STRETCH //
VARIATIONS

These options make stretching this muscle group
more possible with chair assistance and with different positions.

WITH A CHAIR

1. Stand facing away about 1 foot from the seat
of a chair and relax your arms at your sides.

2. Bend your right knee and extend your right leg
backward. Place the top of your right foot flat on
the seat of the chair and push your pelvis
forward. Hold this position for 30 seconds.
(Slightly bend your left knee and slightly lower
yourself for a deeper stretch.) Repeat these
steps with the top of your left foot flat on the
seat of the chair.

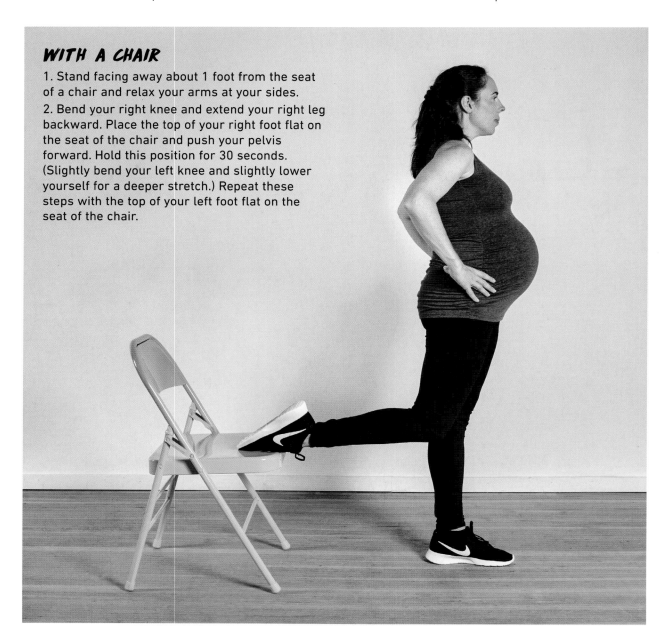

ON YOUR KNEES

1. Place your knees and the tops of your feet flat on the floor. Relax your arms at your sides.

2. Bend your elbows and place your hands flat on your buttocks. Lower your body to place your buttocks on your heels.

3. Slightly lean backward and lift your chin toward the ceiling. Hold this position for 30 seconds.

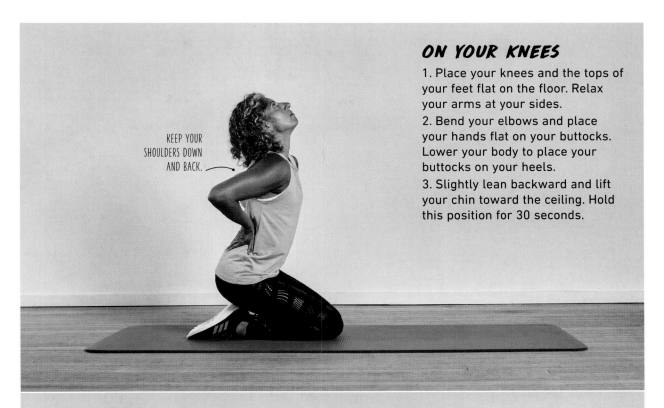

KEEP YOUR SHOULDERS DOWN AND BACK.

ON THE FLOOR

1. Lie on the floor on your left side. Extend your left arm over your head and relax your right arm at your side.

2. Bend your right knee and extend your right leg backward. Grab your right foot with your right hand and push your pelvis forward. Hold this position for 30 seconds. Repeat these steps on your right side and with your left leg extended backward.

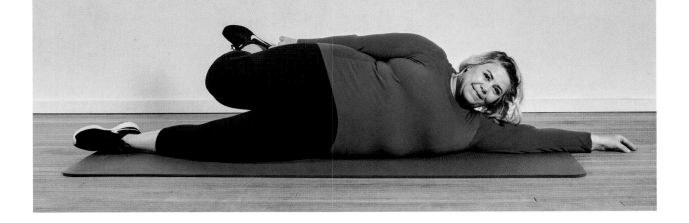

SINGLE-LEG WEIGHT PASS

Whenever your body is off-balance, your brain activates the muscles that improve your ability to control and stabilize the body's position. This exercise challenges your body and mind—and helps bring them into alignment.

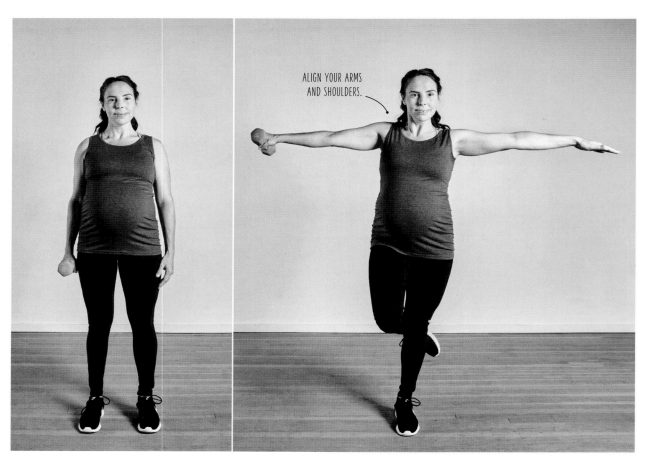

ALIGN YOUR ARMS AND SHOULDERS.

1 Stand with your feet shoulder width apart. Hold a weight in your right hand and relax your arms at your sides.

2 Bend your right knee and place your right foot behind your left calf. Extend your arms toward your sides.

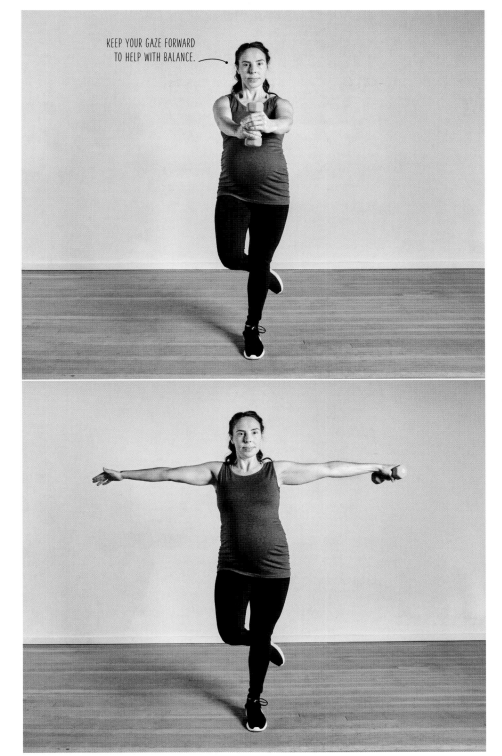

KEEP YOUR GAZE FORWARD
TO HELP WITH BALANCE.

3 Slowly bring your arms toward the middle of your chest. Pass the weight from your right hand to your left hand.

4 Extend your arms toward your sides. Repeat this weight exchange 8 to 10 times. Repeat these steps with your left foot behind your right calf.

// SINGLE-LEG WEIGHT PASS //

VARIATIONS

Your brain needs time to adjust to balance. These quite different modifications will still engage your core and build your balance.

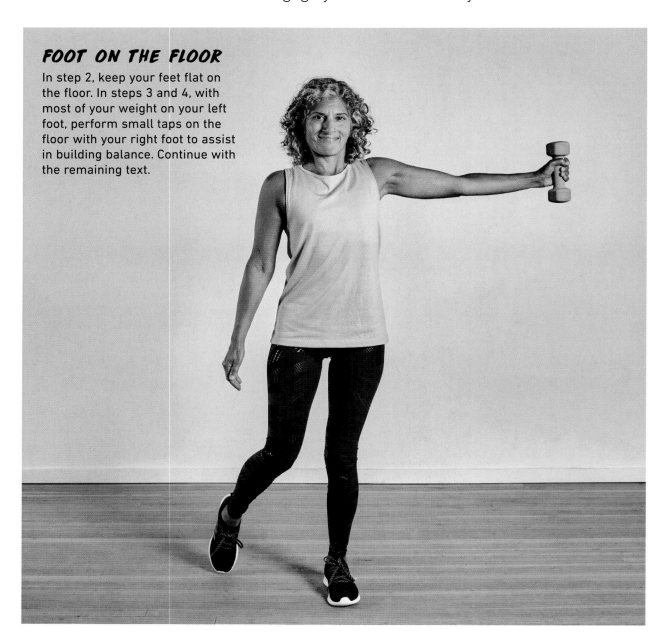

FOOT ON THE FLOOR

In step 2, keep your feet flat on the floor. In steps 3 and 4, with most of your weight on your left foot, perform small taps on the floor with your right foot to assist in building balance. Continue with the remaining text.

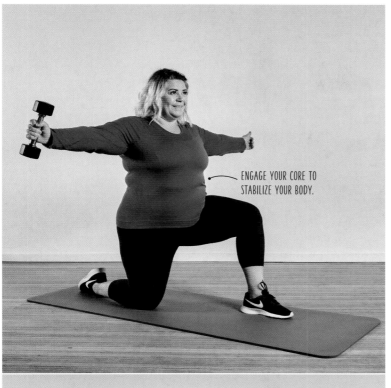

ENGAGE YOUR CORE TO STABILIZE YOUR BODY.

ON ONE KNEE

1. Place your right knee flat on the floor and bend your left knee to place your left foot flat on the floor. Hold a weight in your right hand and extend your arms toward your sides until aligned with your shoulders.

2. Slowly bring your arms toward the middle of your chest. Pass the weight from your right hand to your left hand.

3. Extend your arms toward your sides. Repeat this weight exchange 8 to 10 times. Repeat these steps with your left knee and right foot flat on the floor.

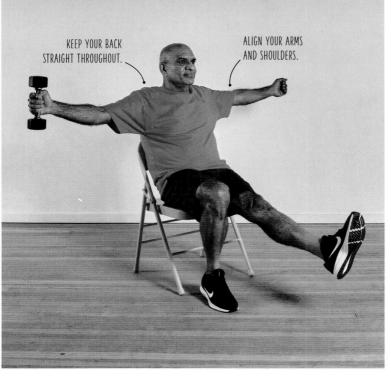

KEEP YOUR BACK STRAIGHT THROUGHOUT.

ALIGN YOUR ARMS AND SHOULDERS.

SEATED

1. Sit in a chair and place your feet flat on the floor. Hold a weight in your right hand and relax your arms at your sides.

2. Lift your left leg until parallel with the floor. Extend your arms toward your sides until aligned with your shoulders.

3. Slowly bring your arms toward the middle of your chest. Pass the weight from your right hand to your left hand.

4. Extend your arms toward your sides. Repeat this weight exchange 8 to 10 times. Repeat these steps with your right leg lifted.

SINGLE-LEG ARM ROTATION

I often train clients in single-leg balance work to build their reactiveness, giving them muscular strength and brain recruitment to prevent falls later in life. These balance exercises are important moves for daily life—now and in the future.

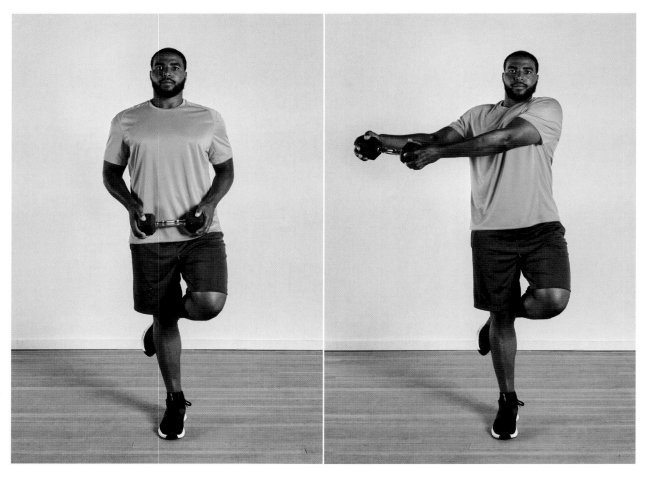

1 Stand with your left foot behind your right calf. Hold one weight in your hands and rest the weight in front of your pelvis.

2 Extend your arms toward your right side until the weight aligns with your chest.

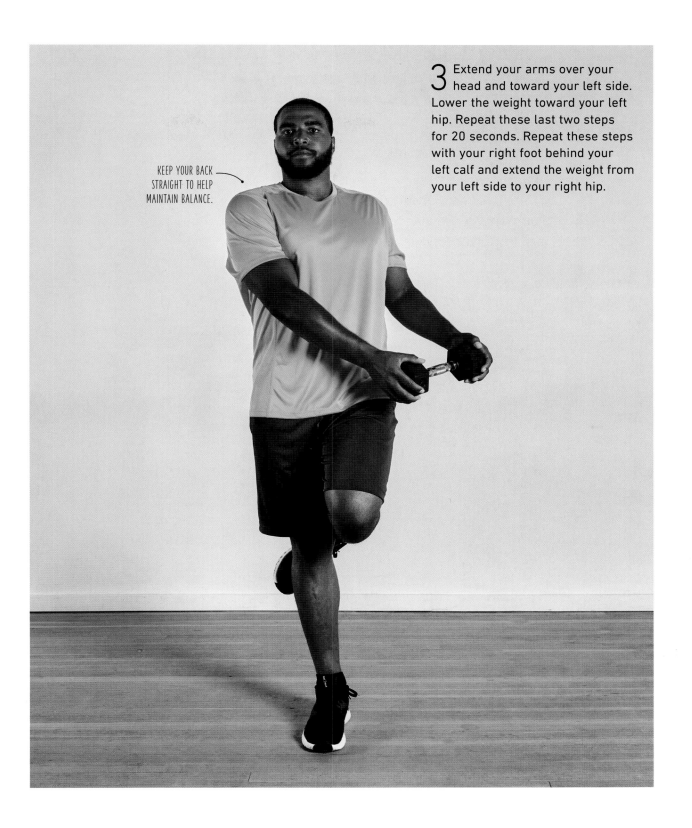

KEEP YOUR BACK STRAIGHT TO HELP MAINTAIN BALANCE.

3 Extend your arms over your head and toward your left side. Lower the weight toward your left hip. Repeat these last two steps for 20 seconds. Repeat these steps with your right foot behind your left calf and extend the weight from your left side to your right hip.

// SINGLE-LEG ARM ROTATION //

VARIATIONS

You can perform this exercise through one of these variations—standing, sitting, or kneeling—to help develop your balance.

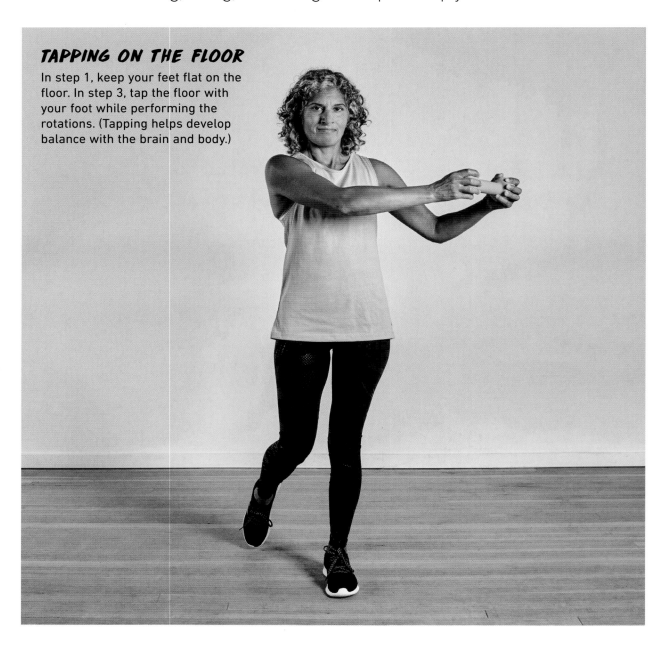

TAPPING ON THE FLOOR

In step 1, keep your feet flat on the floor. In step 3, tap the floor with your foot while performing the rotations. (Tapping helps develop balance with the brain and body.)

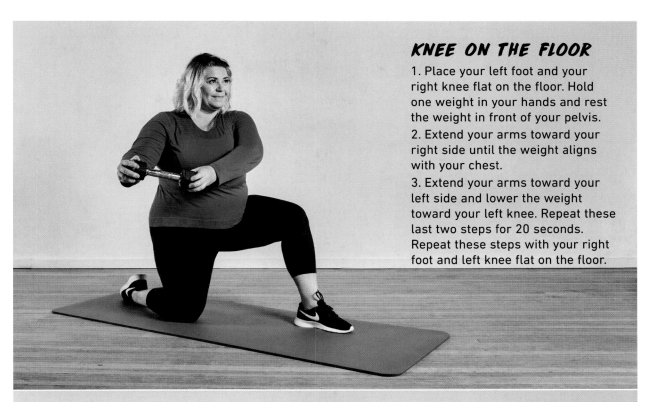

KNEE ON THE FLOOR

1. Place your left foot and your right knee flat on the floor. Hold one weight in your hands and rest the weight in front of your pelvis.
2. Extend your arms toward your right side until the weight aligns with your chest.
3. Extend your arms toward your left side and lower the weight toward your left knee. Repeat these last two steps for 20 seconds. Repeat these steps with your right foot and left knee flat on the floor.

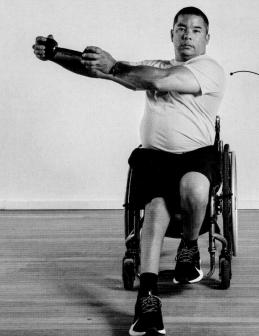

KEEP YOUR SHOULDERS DOWN AND YOUR BACK STRAIGHT THROUGHOUT.

SEATED

In step 1, sit on a chair and place your feet flat on the floor. Continue with the remaining text, but in step 3, extend forward the leg on the same side as the weight.

AIRPLANE

This exercise activates your core stability and balance. Although this isometric exercise requires no movement, holding a position strong—employing your core and glute muscles—can help build muscle endurance.

1 Stand with your feet shoulder width apart and relax your arms at your sides.

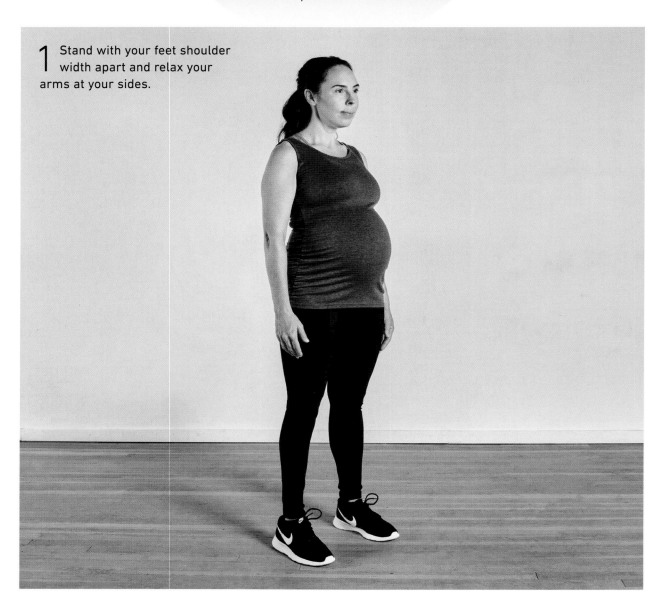

2 Bend at your waist and extend your right leg backward to form a 45-degree angle with your legs. Hold this position for 30 seconds. Repeat these steps with your left leg extended backward.

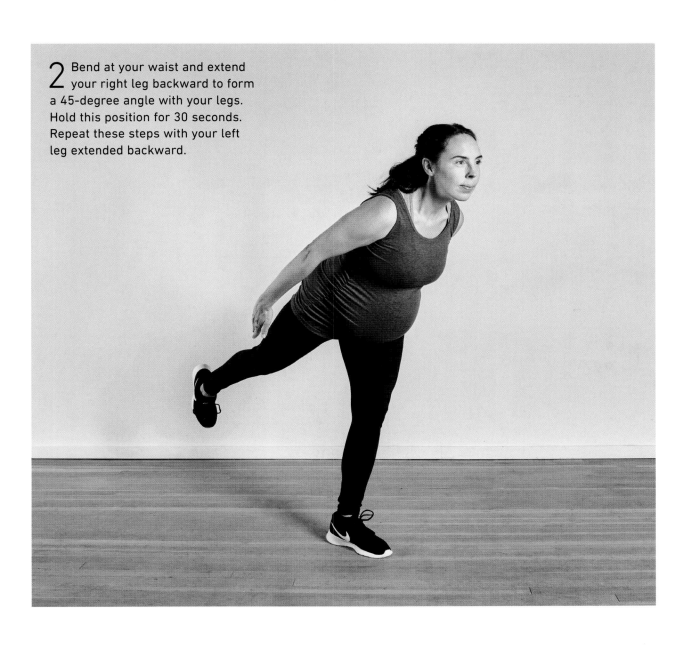

// AIRPLANE //
VARIATIONS

Prepare for takeoff with these helpful variations that offer assistance to your balance with a chair, a wall, or toe taps.

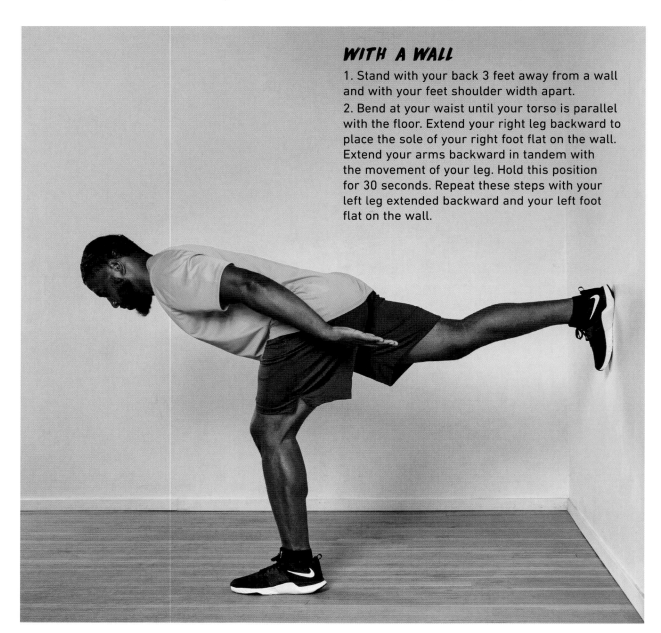

WITH A WALL

1. Stand with your back 3 feet away from a wall and with your feet shoulder width apart.

2. Bend at your waist until your torso is parallel with the floor. Extend your right leg backward to place the sole of your right foot flat on the wall. Extend your arms backward in tandem with the movement of your leg. Hold this position for 30 seconds. Repeat these steps with your left leg extended backward and your left foot flat on the wall.

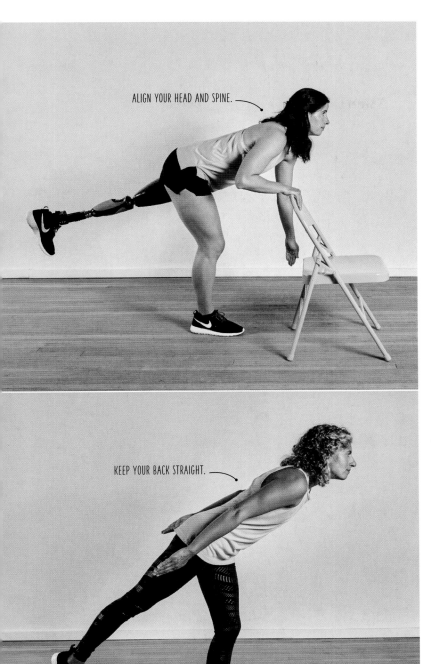

ALIGN YOUR HEAD AND SPINE.

KEEP YOUR BACK STRAIGHT.

WITH A CHAIR

1. Stand behind a chair with your feet shoulder width apart. Place your right hand on the back of the chair and relax your left arm at your side.

2. Bend at your waist and extend your left leg backward until parallel with the floor. Hold this position for 30 seconds. Repeat these steps with your left hand on the back of the chair and your right leg extended backward.

WITH TOE TAPS

In step 2, once you extend your leg backward, intermittently tap the toes of your extended foot on the floor behind you.

PENDULUM

This exercise is an excellent way to work your core and increase your balance. Your goal is to try to stabilize your position between the leg swings. As an added bonus, this exercise also works your quadriceps and glutes with each leg extension.

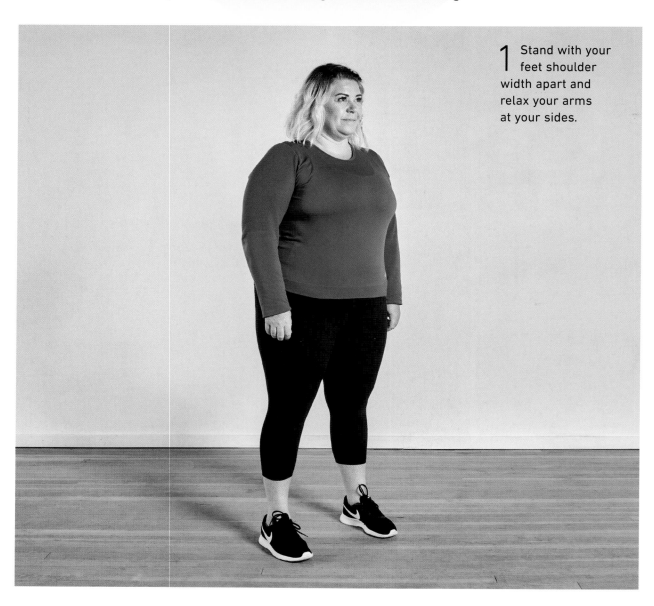

1 Stand with your feet shoulder width apart and relax your arms at your sides.

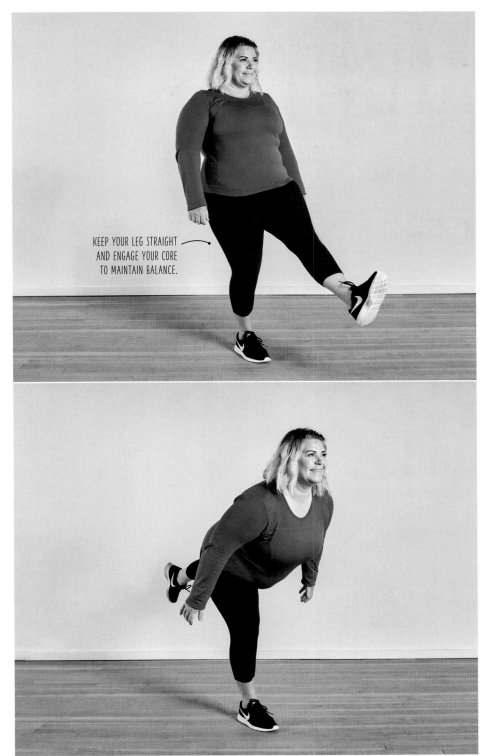

KEEP YOUR LEG STRAIGHT
AND ENGAGE YOUR CORE
TO MAINTAIN BALANCE.

2 Extend your left leg forward until your left foot aligns with your right knee.

3 Slowly swing your left leg backward and bend at your waist. Repeat these last two steps for 30 seconds. Repeat these steps with your right leg.

// PENDULUM //
VARIATIONS

These variations offer balance support with the use of a chair
as well as variety with weights and lateral movements.

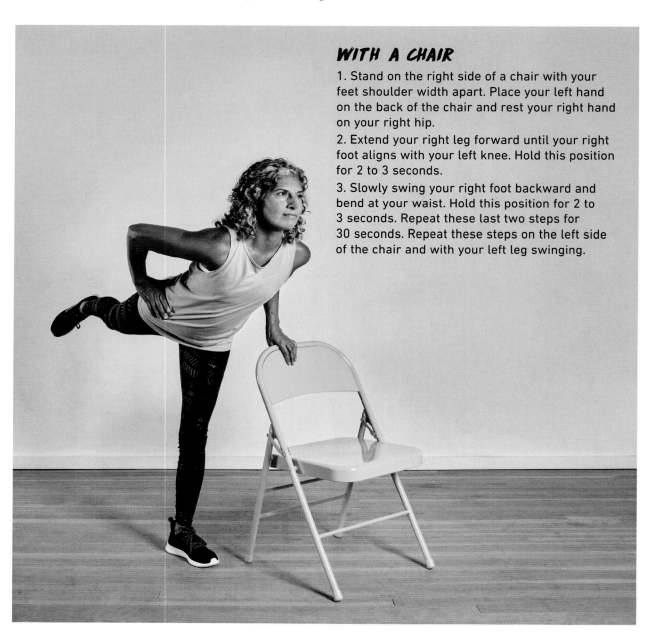

WITH A CHAIR

1. Stand on the right side of a chair with your feet shoulder width apart. Place your left hand on the back of the chair and rest your right hand on your right hip.

2. Extend your right leg forward until your right foot aligns with your left knee. Hold this position for 2 to 3 seconds.

3. Slowly swing your right foot backward and bend at your waist. Hold this position for 2 to 3 seconds. Repeat these last two steps for 30 seconds. Repeat these steps on the left side of the chair and with your left leg swinging.

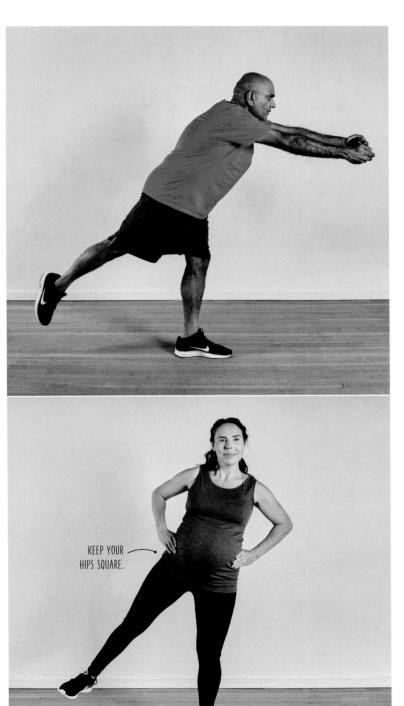

KEEP YOUR HIPS SQUARE.

WITH ONE WEIGHT

1. Stand with your feet shoulder width apart and hold one weight in your hands in front of your chest.

2. Extend your right leg forward and extend your arms forward.

3. Extend your right leg backward. Repeat these last two steps for 30 seconds. Repeat these steps with your left leg extended.

WITH LATERAL MOVEMENTS

1. Stand with your feet shoulder width apart and rest your hands on your hips.

2. Extend your right leg away from your right side. Hold this position for 2 to 3 seconds, then lower your right leg to the floor. Repeat this step 8 to 10 times. Repeat these steps with your left leg extended.

ROB GOSSE

"You're an inspiration" is a phrase I've never felt comfortable with. I prefer to see myself as a father and athlete. I'm no different from anyone else. We all have our own stories. My story just happens to include an accident that changed the way I make my way through the world. I've been an athlete since childhood, and at one time, I was training for the Olympics in gymnastics.

After my accident, I came back to sports—but in the adaptive world. I made it as far as competing in the world competition for disabled waterskiing, setting a Canadian record for my category as well as setting a personal best.

I like to share my story of how sports opened so many doors and opportunities for me that I never thought possible. When I see something and say

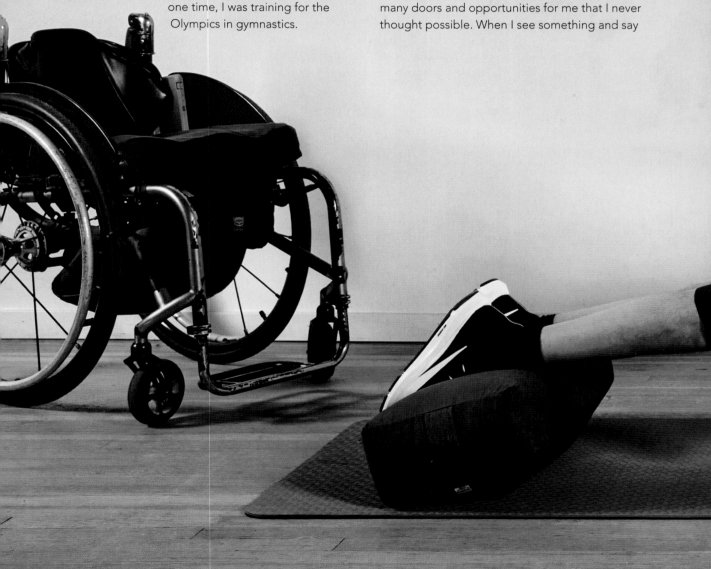

"I want to try that," it's never followed by "but I can't because I have a disability." I try to look at everything through the eyes of "How can I make that work for me?" On the days I just don't have the energy, I lean into my support network to help me see the "how."

My best advice for anyone is to stop telling yourself "I can't" and replace that phrase with "How can I … ?" Just altering the words can change your entire perspective of what you're capable of. As I age, I'm looking for ways to keep my body fit and my brain active. I didn't realize that yoga and basic fitness could be so good at strengthening my muscles. Although my mind will always go for the adrenaline and speed, my physically aging self needs to slow down—just a little but not too much. But no matter my speed, I'm still going to look for the "how."

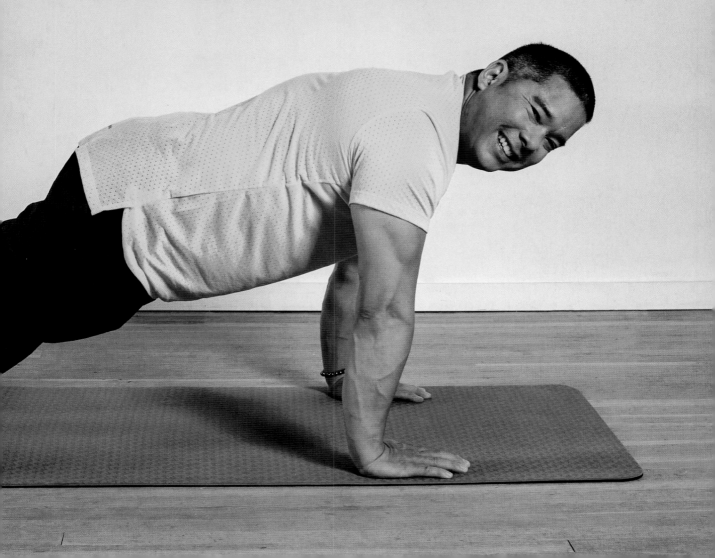

CHAPTER 5
COMBINATIONS, INTERVALS & COMPLEXES

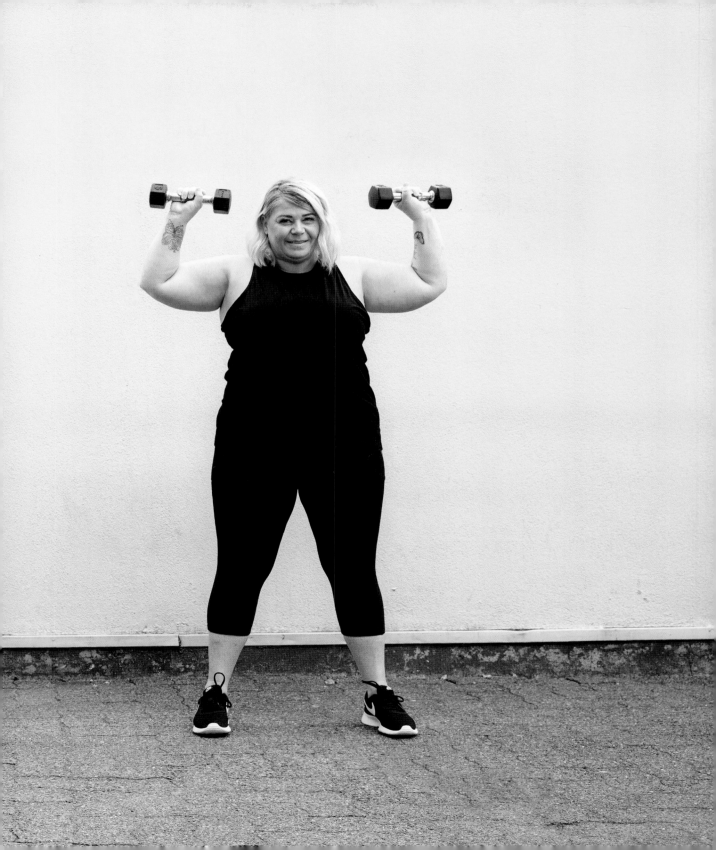

INTERVAL TRAINING
(LONG FORMAT)

This offers a long high-intensity workout. Perform each exercise for 45 seconds and perform this entire set 2 to 3 times.

SPEED SKATING	WOOD CHOP
HIGH KNEES	MOUNTAIN CLIMBER
PUSH-UP	JAB & CROSS
SQUAT KICK	BURPEE
LATERAL LEG RAISE	SINGLE-LEG CALF RAISE

INTERVAL TRAINING
(SHORT FORMAT)

This offers a short high-intensity workout. Perform each exercise for 30 seconds and perform this entire set 2 to 3 times.

BICEPS CURL	JAB & CROSS
T-RAISE	PENDULUM
FAST FEET	V-SIT OBLIQUE ROTATION
SQUAT	JUMPING JACK
DEADLIFT	AIRPLANE

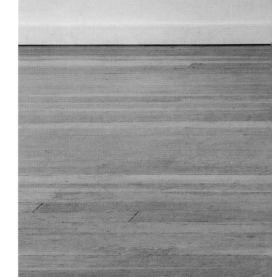

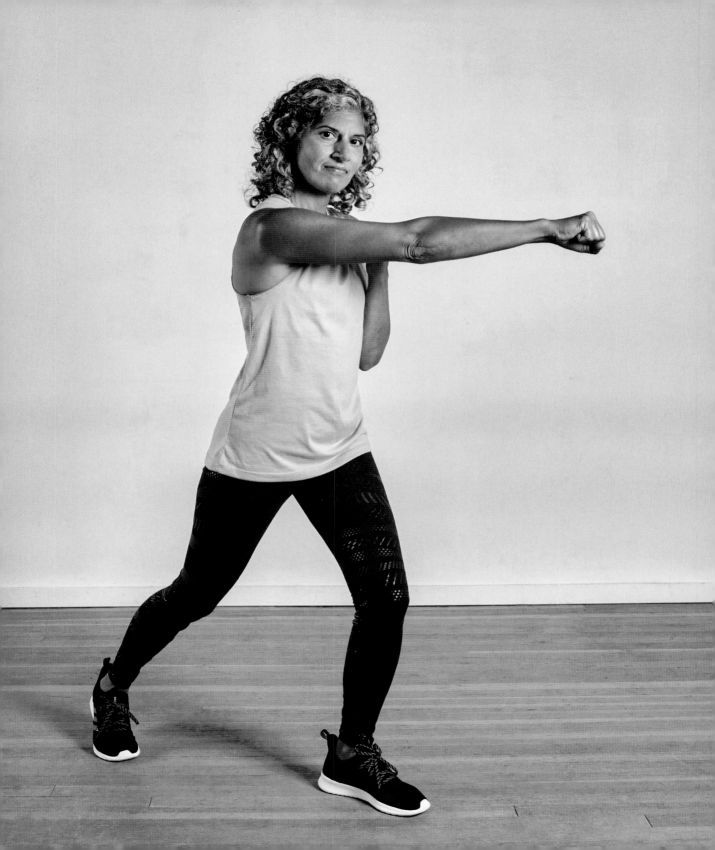

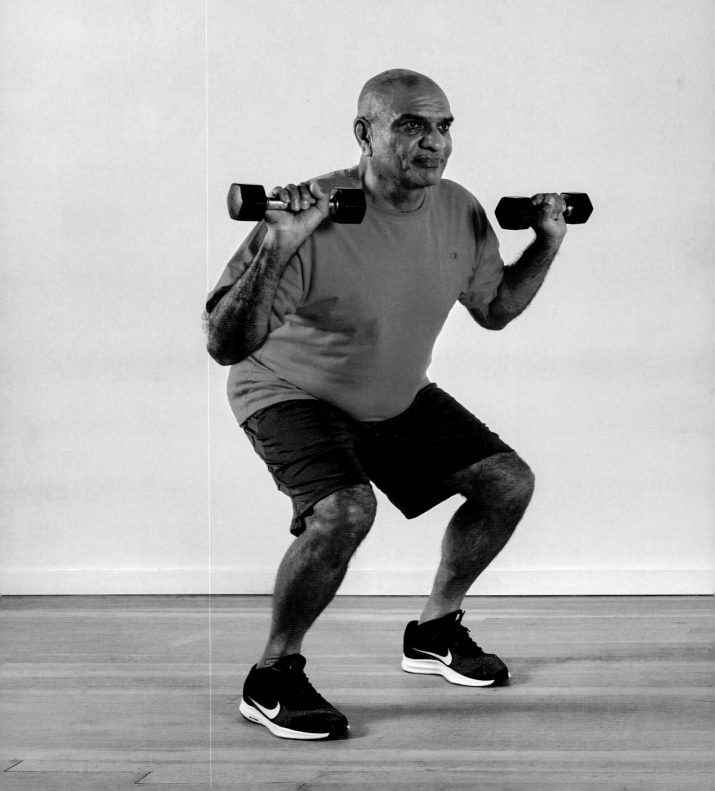

MULTI-ACTION
(LONG FORMAT)

These exercises include more than one muscle group in each move.
Perform each exercise for 45 seconds and perform this entire set 2 to 3 times.

SQUAT TO SHOULDER PRESS	BURPEE
SPEED SKATING	WOOD CHOP
BICEPS CURL CROSSOVER	SUPERHERO
HIP THRUST	SPLIT STANCE FRONT RAISE
SINGLE-LEG WEIGHT PASS	PENDULUM

MULTI-ACTION
(SHORT FORMAT)

These exercises also include more than one muscle group in each move.
Perform each exercise for 30 seconds and perform this entire set 2 to 3 times.

SINGLE-LEG ARM ROTATION	LEG DROP
SQUAT KICK	REVERSE LUNGE
DEAD BUG	LATERAL LEG RAISE
SQUAT TO SHOULDER PRESS	BICEPS CURL
SIDE PLANK	AIRPLANE

FULL-BODY COMPLEX (LONG FORMAT)

These exercises give you a longer full-body workout. Perform each exercise for 45 seconds and perform this entire set 2 to 3 times.

PULLOVER

TRICEPS DIP

WALL SIT

GLUTE & LEG EXTENSION

UPRIGHT PLANK

BENT-OVER ROW

PUSH-UP

DONKEY KICK

SQUAT

SUPERHERO

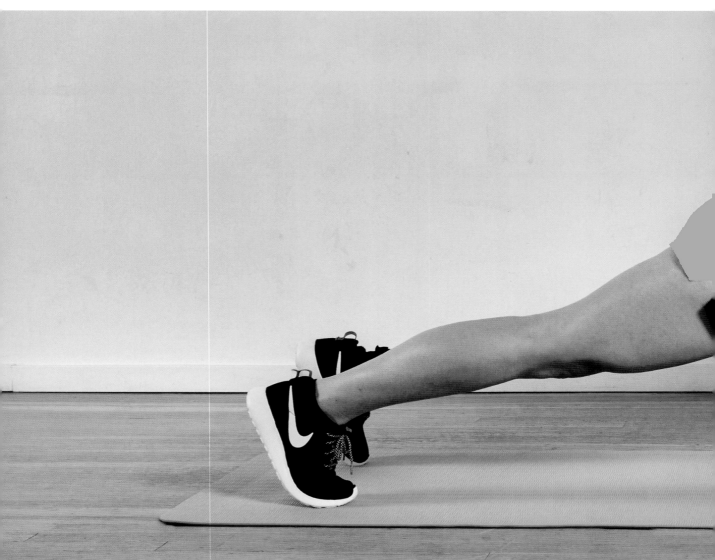

FULL-BODY COMPLEX (SHORT FORMAT)

These exercises give you a shorter full-body workout when time is limited. Perform each exercise for 45 seconds and perform this entire set 2 to 3 times.

DEAD BUG

SINGLE-LEG WEIGHT PASS

CHEST PRESS

SQUAT TO SHOULDER PRESS

TRIANGLE PUSH-UP

DEADLIFT

BICEP CURLS

T-RAISE

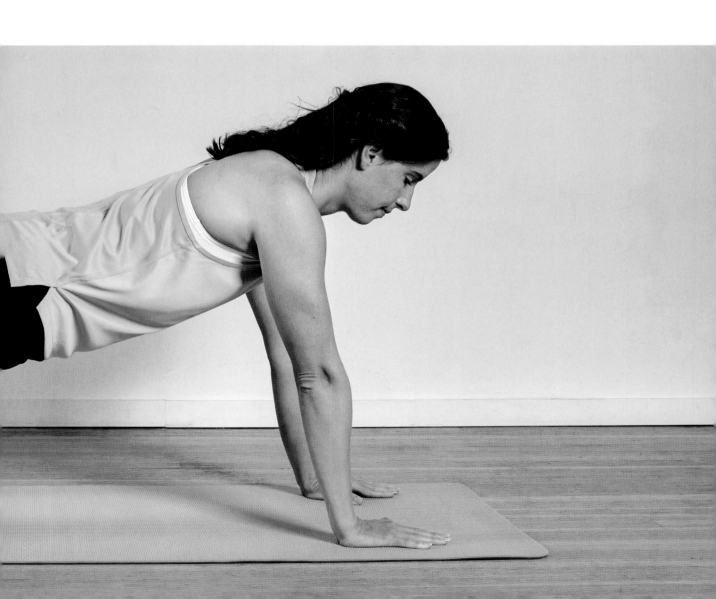

STRETCH & BALANCE COMPLEXES

These exercises can help with balance development.
Perform each exercise for 30 seconds,
then switch to the opposite side (where applicable).

HAMSTRING STRETCH

CALF STRETCH

AIRPLANE

QUAD STRETCH

HIP FLEXOR STRETCH

GLUTE MEDIUS STRETCH

OBLIQUE & LAT STRETCH

CHEST & PECTORAL STRETCH

SHOULDER STRETCH

UPPER BACK STRETCH

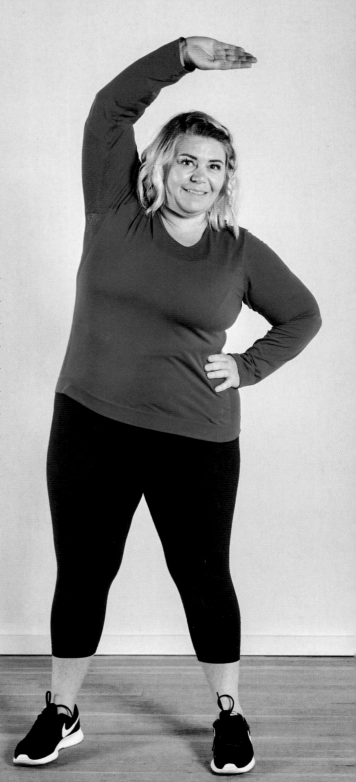

UPPER BODY

These exercises are dedicated to your upper body.
Perform each exercise for 30 seconds
and perform this entire set 2 to 3 times.

PUSH-UP

LAT PULLDOWN

BICEPS CURL

T-RAISE

PULLOVER

CHEST PRESS

TRICEPS DIP

BENT-OVER ROW

UPRIGHT PULL

SPLIT STANCE FRONT RAISE

LOWER BODY

These exercises are dedicated to your lower body.
Perform each exercise for 30 seconds
and perform this entire set 2 to 3 times.

HIP THRUST

DONKEY KICK

SQUAT

HIGH KNEES

REVERSE LUNGE

SINGLE-LEG CALF RAISE

LATERAL LEG RAISE

WALL SIT

FAST FEET

DEADLIFT

CORE

These exercises are dedicated to core strength.
Perform each exercise for 30 seconds
and perform this entire set 2 to 3 times.

V-SIT OBLIQUE ROTATION	LEG DROP
DEAD BUG	WOOD CHOP
SUPERHERO	SIDE PLANK
AIRPLANE	PENDULUM
SINGLE-LEG WEIGHT PASS	SINGLE-LEG ARM ROTATION

INDEX

ABOUT THE AUTHOR

Louise Green is a celebrated author, influencer, and award-winning fitness trainer who has been changing the narrative of our fitness culture since 2007. Her passion is to lead people to find their inner athlete at every size, age, and ability, accumulating more than 10,000 hours specializing in size-inclusive fitness while working toward a fitness culture that's accessible for all.

She's the founder of Big Fit Girl—now a brand, a fitness app, a book, a weekly podcast, and a monthly magazine column at *SELF* magazine. Her work has impacted thousands of people from around the globe and encouraged them to step off the sidelines. Louise is the first plus-size athlete to be featured by *Triathlete*, *Bicycling*, *Impact*, *Strong*, and *Runner's World UK* magazines.

Her unique approach to inclusive fitness has landed her many accolades: She's been named one of the top trainers to follow by *SELF*; one of "Eight Badass Women Who Prove Fitness Has No Size" by *People* magazine; one of "Sixty Barbie Role Models Positively Impacting Girls" by Mattel; one of the "Top 100 Health and Fitness Influencers" by *Optimyz* magazine (three years in a row); and one of "5 Canadian Women Boldly Changing the World for Women and Girls" by *Women of Influence*.

Louise has previously authored two books and has been featured by more than 150 media outlets, including the *Steve Harvey Show*, the *Australian Morning Show*, and London's *This Morning*. She's also been featured in many national brand campaigns, helping hone the message that fitness, beauty, and confidence have no size. She tenaciously works toward making "fitness for everyone" a daily reality.

ACKNOWLEDGMENTS

Writing this book was such an amazing opportunity for me to share my passion for inclusive and accessible fitness. I'd like to thank my first running coach, Chris, for showing me that all bodies have the possibility to shine like an athlete if given the right tools and encouragement. I'd also like to thank all my clients over the years—you've been my best teachers—and my associate, Tarryn, for always being behind the scenes helping to make this happen. Finally, I'd like to thank Christopher Stolle at DK Publishing for trusting in me and giving me the opportunity to write this book.